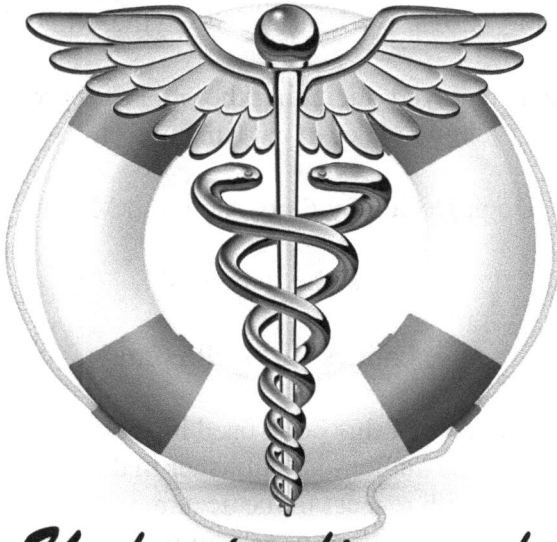

Understanding and
SURVIVING
Obamacare

James W. Forsythe, MD, HMD

Understanding and Surviving Obamacare

Century Wellness Publishing

Book Design by Patty Atcheson Melton

Forsythe, James W.

1. Politics 2. Health Care

ISBN: 978-09897636-0-8

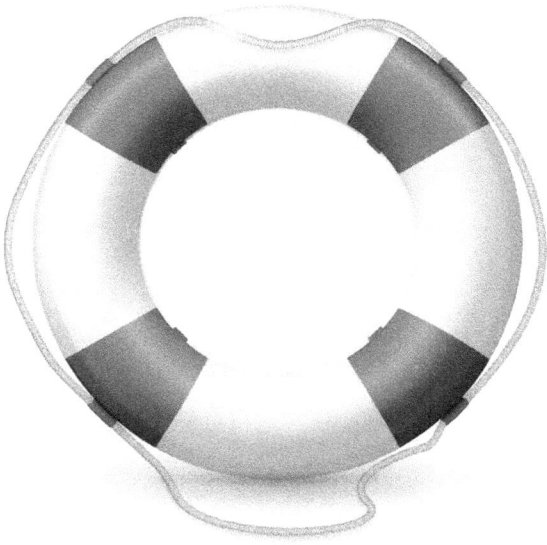

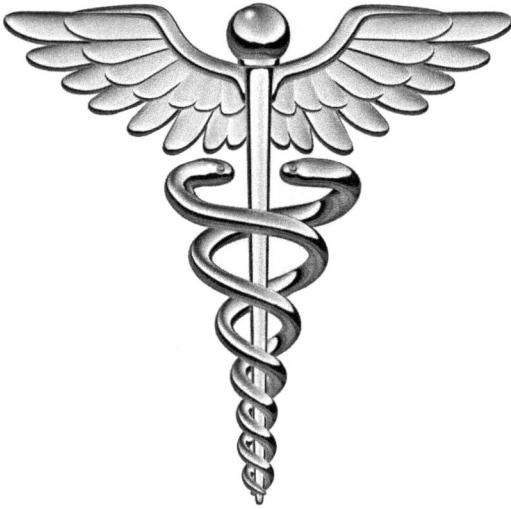

Dedication

To the many countless people nationwide who have couragously admitted their serious mistake of initially supporting Obamacare ~ now proclaiming that the legislation will harm virtually all Americans. This book would not have been possible with the support, dedication and commitment of my intelligent and prophetic wife, Earlene Forsythe who has understood perhaps better than anyone of the horrors that Obamacare imposes on all Americans--unless repealed or revised. Earlene is among many dedicated friends and patients who have continuously encouraged me to press forward with the development of this vital publication.

Contents

Foreword

Just about everyone involved acknowledged that the coming "train wreck" would soon occur.

Yes, politicians from both sides of the aisle started predicting this outcome for Obamacare starting in the spring of 2013.

As many Americans now know, this massive proverbial locomotive accident occurred on schedule stating October 1, 2013.

That's precisely when the destruction of the USA's medical and health insurance industries commenced, on time and reliably as planned primarily by the liberals in Congress working with President Barack Obama.

Starting that week, countless millions of people got put on hold when calling for help signing up for the Affordable Health Care Act, or they got a "404 default" hang-up notice upon attempting to access the inept U.S. and state government Obamacare Websites.

Sadly, as the costs to build and maintain the faulty online systems approached $1 billion, President Obama claimed the Web issue could be quickly fixed.

These were mighty tall words, considering the fact that the guy and his bureaucrats had nearly 3 ½ years to build the Obamacare Websites and the related consumer call-in system.

"What?" I thought upon hearing of his statements. "This guy can't be serious. Are people across America going to believe his hogwash?"

Sure enough, as my many years of intense research shows as described in the following pages, if left unchecked Obamacare will wreak havoc on our nation's economy while steadily dismantling the efficiency of America's health care system.

Indeed, while acknowledging the fact that Obama and his socialist cronies can't build a mere Website, just imagine the steadily worsening damage that their deranged policies will do to us all—upon obliterating the efficiency and the competitiveness of the U.S. health care system.

The same bureaucratic administrators unable to generate and manage contractors and staffers in building basic links on Websites—angering millions of people—are now being put in charge of managing all of our health care decisions.

Whether Democrats and even some Republicans want to admit this or not, without exaggeration the issue comes down to the fact that a warped, over-the-top ideology is forcing all Americans to get a system that most of them do not want.

Worsening matters, the Obamacare administration ignored the passionate pleas of growing numbers of liberal newspapers that eventually called for the act to be nullified and rewritten.

The steady stream of anti-Obamacare commentary swelled starting in the spring of 2013, with the liberal "Washington Post" and "New York Times"—boosted by similar commentary from the "Chicago Tribune"—helped to lead the anti-Obamacare mindset.

To their credit, by mid-2013 those same newspapers and many others admitted they had been "wrong" when originally supporting the misguided legislation when first passed by Congress in March 2010.

Meantime, also during the first half of 2013 many labor unions that formerly helped champion the Act's original passage also withdrew their support for this misguided law.

Sadly however, steeped in their selfish philosophies and warped political ideology, Obama and the Democrats in Congress turned their backs on the will of a vast majority of Americans—allowing the first major nationwide phase of Obamacare to begin as scheduled with the wretched and useless Website.

Streams of shocked Americans then discovered that their mandatory insurance premiums had skyrocketed to unaffordable levels. Just as disturbing, countless thousands of Americans felt shocked upon learning their insurance had been dropped.

From that point forward, the many negative triggering points clicked into gear, issues that I first noticed and started telling many people about as soon as Obama was first elected in October 2008.

Mindful of these many pitfalls, every American has a right to know the truth, regarding each destructive phase of Obamacare that scheduled to click into gear on a pre-planned time schedule throughout the remainder of this, the second decade of the 21st Century.

The undeniable, irrefutable facts regarding Obamacare that I list in the pages that follow should shock and disturb every thoughtful, intelligent American.

As you'll soon discover, without the repeal of Obamacare or an extensive revamp of the Act, the spending power of all individual Americans will decrease substantially—while millions of citizens get forced off of health insurance rolls.

Anyone who ignores or who refuses to acknowledge these disturbing and destructive issues shall become doomed to potential financial destruction—coupled with the a critical degradation in health care services.

--James W. Forsythe, M.D., H.M.D.

Although now having health insurance through their employers, many of the 250 million hard-working U.S. citizens with jobs may soon lose their coverage.

1

Disturbing Facts on Obamacare

Penalties: Any adult without medical insurance in the United States starting in January 2014 will face fines that over time could reach up to several thousand dollars.

Job losses: Tens of thousands or perhaps even millions of Americans will lose their health insurance via their employers.

Political incompetence: Most members of the U.S. Senate and the U.S. House of Representatives voted on the 2,572-page legislation without reading the bill.

A stark reality strikes many Americans once they learn these grim facts. Obamacare will never be repealed or updated any time in the near future.

The re-election of President Barack Obama and the Democrat-controlled Senate will block any repeal or the adoption of any significant changes.

Although now having health insurance through their employers, many of the 250 million hard-working U.S. citizens with jobs may soon lose their coverage.

The Patient Protection and Affordable Care Act, enacted by Congress in March 2010, commonly referred to as "Obamacare," had the worthy goal of expanding health insurance to Americans unable to afford such coverage.

Sadly however, these regulations will wreak havoc on the entire U.S. health care industry, which had been experiencing a severe recession when Congress enacted law.

Instead, the new rules authorize the inept government to assume control of your health care; and drastically lower the quality of healthcare services that patients receive.

Finally aware of Obamacare's many pitfalls, in the first several months of 2013 many labor unions started strikes or threatened walkouts due to hot-button issues stemming from the legislation. Among just a handful of these developments:

Wall Street Journal: "Union leaders say many of the law's requirements will drive up the cost of their health-care plans and make unionized workers less competitive." Also noted by the "Journal," Obamacare eliminates medical benefits caps that some employer-provided health insurance plans had been providing and the elimination of price limits on certain drugs that some employers had used as cost-containment measures. "To offset that, the nation's largest labor groups want their lower-paid members to be able to get federal insurance subsidies while remaining on their plans."

Jackson Free Press: Mississippi emerged as one of numerous states where politicians continued to voice their opposition to the Act's requirement that individual states create online-based exchanges where customers can shop for health-care plans. As reported by the Jackson, Mississippi, newspaper in February 2013, that state's insurance commissioner, Mike Chaney, had been working the previous three years to develop the Magnolia State's exchange. However, the U.S. Department of Health and Human Services rejected the state's proposed exchange, noting that Gov. Phil Bryant had a stated "intent to oppose implementation of the state-based exchange."

Real Clear Politics: An article by Ben Domenech said that federal officials within the Congressional Budget Office (CBO), a non-partisan agency that forecasts and analyzes spending and revenues of the U.S. government, voiced their concerns regarding the implementation of Obamacare. Among the most serious issues they cited: Updated estimates project that Obamacare subsidies through state-run insurance exchanges will surpass $1 trillion through 2022, up from the previous estimate of $814 billion; the re-calculated totals estimate that average exchange subsidies will skyrocket to $5,510 in 2014 when Obamacare starts—up from the previous estimate of $3,970, a total that had been calculated for that year when Congress passed the Act.

Updated report: An additional "Wall Street Journal" report, as cited in the Real Clear Politics article, noted that as of August 2012, the CBO had estimated that through 2022 four million people would be dropped by their employers from employer-paid health insurance coverage. By February 2013, the CBO's previous estimate increased 75 percent to seven million people. The drop of employees from employer-paid programs is expected because workers will have new options to buy coverage on their own. The estimate suddenly changed because Congress reached a "fiscal cliff" deal that refrained from implementing any significant cuts in federal spending and stopping potential tax increases on the middle class.

Concluding remarks: In ending his report summarizing the CBO's latest findings, Domenech stated that: "Taken together, this is a report that shows how already Obamacare is failing to match the hopes of its creators in many respects. Expect this trend to continue in future years. There is going to be a lot of political fractiousness and market disruption over a policy which may ultimately end up nudging the insured percentage only slightly."

Chapter 1
Summary

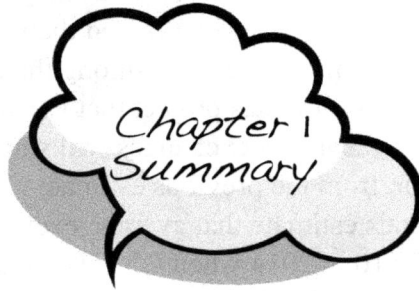

Obamacare will obliterate and ravage the U.S. economy while weakening the health care business. Meantime, citizens will be fined if they refuse to buy insurance policies, even if they prefer to avoid getting such products. The confusion began even as Obama's second four-year term started, when labor unions that previously supported Obamacare began to realize the Act's many pitfalls.

2
Disturbing Facts on Obamacare

Projected layoffs: Streams of health care professionals and especially nurses will face layoffs as Obamacare slashes federal spending on what hospitals receive to care for certain patients—particularly senior citizens.

Growing bureaucracy: Thousands of new agents employed by the IRS will start harassing taxpayers starting in 2014, when citizens must begin proving that they have federally mandated personal health insurance.

Goofy and ridiculous rules: Complicated and confusing new regulations required by Obamacare mean that health insurance policies that many Americans had before 2014 no longer would meet the federal government's puzzling rules.

Political Corruption

Streams of politicians have lied to or misled the public about Obamacare, particularly over-the-top liberals like House Minority leader Nancy Pelosi, a Democrat representing the San Francisco Bay Area.

The Congressional Budget Office reports that the U.S. federal budget deficit continues to skyrocket to the upper stratosphere after surpassing $16 trillion.

Yet in February 2012 Pelosi had the gall to tell Chris Wallace of Fox News that she does not believe the U.S. government has a spending problem.

Reckless comments and extreme political ideologies such as Pelosi's threaten the fabric of the American economy. These political wimps refuse to acknowledge the findings of economics experts from the Heritage Foundation.

The congresswoman and her liberal allies promote reckless Obamacare rules and bloated federal spending, while refusing to address essential spending cuts.

Critical Answers About Obamacare

You must comply with stringent and irrational regulations by providing proof of your insurance coverage when filing your taxes. These mandatory regulations begin January 1, 2014. The initial fine against violators can include the withholding of any refund that might be due to them. Fines in subsequent years will climb to hundreds or thousands of dollars per violator. The specific amount of each penalty will depend on which calendar year a violation occurred, coupled with the individual's income level.

Taxpayers whose employers drop their insurance coverage or who have not already had such policies on their own will be forced to enter mandatory systems. People and their families supposedly will have the ability to make these decisions. But their choices will be limited. Those who meet low-income eligibility requirements can enter the under-funded federal Medicaid program. Whether they want to or not, the other option will force the remaining people not already covered by employer-funded insurance to choose from among policies listed on state health exchanges where policies have been approved by government bureaucrats.

The government-sanctioned insurance exchanges will drastically lower the quality of health care. In essence, the insurance exchanges are the equivalent of multiplex movie theater complexes that offer tickets to just one movie. The show offered to consumers never changes. As a result, all consumers choosing policies from the exchanges will have no choice other than to choose a one-size-fits-all policy.

While stifling competition among health care facilities, the new rules will force the federal government to start paying hundreds of billions of dollars less to hospitals for the care of seniors. Even before the policy mandate was to take effect at the beginning of 2014, these rules started a negative "trickle-down" effect. Decreased budgets caused by the cutbacks forced hospitals to assign nurses to a sharply increased number of patients. This damaged the overall quality of patient care. Nurses from various communities started calling strikes.

The overall quality of health care services will decrease from levels of the past. Health insurance companies will benefit largely because healthy people will be forced to purchase one-size-fits-all policies. This will cut down on competition among health care providers, which will lose their motivation to provide the best services possible.

People with pre-existing negative health conditions will benefit because insurance companies no longer will be able to bar them from getting policies. By being required to purchase policies, healthy people essentially will be forced to cover the bill for patients suffering from pre-existing negative health conditions.

People who benefit will include drug abusers whose bodies and brains get ravaged by their addictions and even narcotics distributors shot in turf wars. Conversely, law-abiding, non-addicted individuals must pay while others essentially "get a free ride." Although many Obamacare supporters want to say otherwise, the facts here prove these socialized health care advocates "wrong." In essence, law abiding citizens with government-approved health insurance will be covering the medical bills of narcotics pushers and drug abusers who either refuse to or fail to get such policies.

Chapter 2 Summary

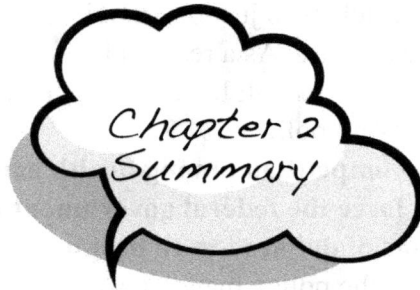

The overall quality of health care in the United States will deteriorate, while certain lawbreakers get a free ride on health care coverage and medical industry professionals get locked in heated labor disputes. The American public will suffer overall. Insurance policy premium fees will increase while the quality of health care services plummets.

3

Inept Regulations Will Destroy Health Care

Sloppy regulations: The mindless regulations will gradually force many union represented people who now have good health insurance to buy substandard policies.

Oversight: The federal government will carefully monitor your doctors' decisions regarding your health, to ensure that those choices comply with federal regulations.

Dropped coverage: By some estimates a whopping one out of three employers will consider dropping employee policies due to soaring costs.

Wrong Choices for Americans

People who have never even been interested in politics will soon discover the disturbing truth that the U.S. government is encroaching on their lives due to Obamacare.

Some politicians including Congresswoman Pelosi have admitted that many representatives never even read Obamacare's many provisions before approving the law.

Due largely to the inept overall performance of Congress, Americans who have not already learned about Obamacare's many intrusions on their lives are about to discover streams of disturbing facts. Among them:

Embracing socialist policies on the verge of communism, for the first time in history our corrupt government will manipulate how doctors treat patients—even if those individuals have private insurance policies. Sadly, as stipulated by certain sections of the law, the Secretary of Health and Human Services will have the power to determine what doctors are authorized to do in treating specific medical conditions. The federal government will be putting handcuffs on doctors, often preventing physicians from administering specialized treatments geared to your unique medical conditions.

Playing politics rather than ruling on the constitutional merits of the law or using common sense, the U.S. Supreme Court has cleared a pathway for these demonic changes. Many of them based in Washington, D.C., far from where most Americans live, bureaucrats are essentially being given carte blanch to essentially "play with" or to manipulate your health care coverage in whatever way they deem fit. Worsening matters, in most cases the government paper pushers have absolutely no medical training or experience in the health care field.

Countless detrimental changes are on tap, poised to negatively impact your personal finances, your job and your home life. The specifics listed here thus far are just a handful of the many hundreds of Obamacare regulations poised to negatively impact the lives of Americans. By some accounts, the average person would need several months to thoroughly read, absorb and understand the initial 2,572 pages of the Obamacare bill that Congress eventually made law. In addition, tens of thousands of "policy pages" regarding Obamacare reportedly have been crafted by various federal agencies since Congress enacted the law.

Chapter 3 Summary

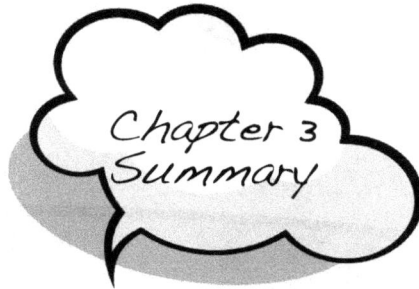

The original provisions of the Obamacare Act and policies subsequently generated by many federal agencies are so voluminous that no single individual understands or "knows" everything about the regulations. Law-abiding taxpayers and their families who have authorized health care policies will essentially be forced to pay for the coverage of drug addicts and heroin or cocaine pushers who fail to or refuse to obtain such coverage. Middle-income and high-income Americans will be forced to pay for the healthcare of people who illegally entered the United States. Those benefiting most without having to pay a single penny will include "illegal aliens" unable to qualify for Medicaid, Medicare or government subsidies for their own insurance. Hard-working people will be required to fund the health care of people who suffer severe medical conditions as a result of their own reckless and lawless behavior. The federal government will "handcuff" doctors into giving only specific types of coverage for certain medical conditions. These rules will prevent physicians from implementing treatments for unique ailments, diseases or injuries. Much of the time, the government-mandated treatment criteria will be imposed by people with absolutely no medical training or health industry experience.

Squeezing low-income and middle-class Americans, the IRS began imposing a 3.8 percent unearned income taz and a Medicare Part A payroll tax.

4

The Destructive Obamacare Timetable Clicks into Gear

Destruction looms: The many dangerous provisions of Obamacare are set to click into gear in pre-determined phases through the second decade of the 21ˢᵗ Century.

Congressional ignorance: The vast majority of congressmen and senators have little if any notion on the many specific destructive requirements imposed by the Act.

Costs skyrocket: Federal funding for Obamacare will more than double by 2020 as the government solidifies methods of requiring doctors to administer treatments in "authorized ways"— as mandated by politicians and bureaucrats.

March 2010

Congress narrowly enacted the Patient Protection and Affordable Care Act although many congressmen and senators had never read the bill. President Obama quickly signed the legislation into law, over-eager to enact reckless legislation. Lawsuits filed by more than 20 states sought to eliminate the new regulations under the grounds that the forced-mandate to buy policies was unconstitutional.

July 2010

Streams of Obamacare tax hikes mandated by the law started, such as fees on tanning salons.

September 2010

Guaranteed a high probability of profits due to provisions that force healthy people to buy policies, the nation's private insurance companies began implementing various required provisions. Among them:

Co-pays: Consumers and companies buying heath insurance policies were forced to start paying for preventative care in their premiums, a change that gradually started eliminating co-pay structures for certain healthcare checkups.

Young adults: The new rules enabled parents of young adults through their mid-20s to remain on their parents' health care policies.

Eliminate: The update prohibited insurance companies from continuing to sell "mini-med plans" that had capped the total amounts that could be paid for specific care.

January 2011

Armed with a new provision that enabled them to increase the federal bureaucracy, the government started imposing new penalties on Health Savings Accounts. Additional provisions that ultimately will pump up consumer healthcare costs clicked into gear when the government started slapping new taxes on pharmaceutical companies, plus the manufacturers and distributors of medical devices.

June 2012

In perhaps one of its most controversial rulings of the past century, the U.S. Supreme court on a narrow 5-to-4 vote declared as constitutional most of Obamacare. The same rulings authorized individual states to decide whether they will expand Medicaid in accordance with the Act's overall national strategy.

January 2013

Squeezing low-income and middle-class Americans, the IRS

began imposing a 3.8 percent unearned income tax and a Medicare Part A payroll tax.

January 2014

Americans will start paying penalties unless they have government-authorized health insurance policies, particularly individuals or families not already on Medicaid or Medicare. Slapping American industry and potentially forcing many small firms out of business, companies with at least 50 employees must pay penalties if the firms fail to provide health insurance for employees.

January 2018

According to some news reports, the federally mandated Independent Payment Advisory Board (IPAB,) a bureaucratic panel with no required medical training and which reports to Congress, will begin slashing health care budgeting geared for seniors. The federal government starts penalizing high-end health care plans that people buy for themselves, imposing what some observers call a "Cadillac tax."

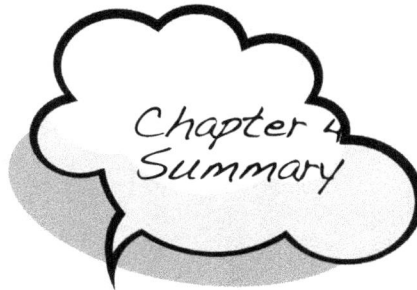

Chapter 4 Summary

The financial pain suffered by American consumers and taxpayers will steadily intensify in pre-designated phases through the second decade of the 21st Century. Consumer costs will steadily increase as the various bureaucratic provisions of Obamacare click into gear on a pre-scheduled timetable.

"If you think theft is a problem now, wait until Uncle Sam serves up critical information on 300 million American citizens on a platter."

5

Personal Privacy Obliterted

Privacy: Doctors from all major specialties will be having instant access to your private medical information.

Data: Streams of government agencies will get the ability to snoop into your personal health care data.

Security nightmare: Some bureaucrats propose laws that will enable you to determine who has checked your health care records—but only "after the fact."

Big Government Will Manage Your Life

When considering the federal government's awesome power to delve into your personal health records, nightmarish visions of George Orwell's classic futuristic mid-20th Century novel "1984" come to mind.

As an example of the power that Obamacare will have to wreck your life, consider the case of former New York congressman Anthony Weiner. The lawmaker resigned in June 2011 at the height of a sex scandal.

Amid his political downfall the congressman announced that he was seeking treatment for sexual addiction. Due to Obamacare, such records on all Americans will become available to any doctor that a person visits.

Thus, a person treated as a young adult for mental illness

would have those records reviewed in his mid-60s by a dentist that he visits. As a result, the potential to destroy a person's reputation will surge due to Obamacare's open-book regulations.

"Your oral surgeon doesn't need to know about your erectile dysfunction or your bout with depression 20 years ago," the "New York Post" said in June 2011. "Nevertheless, such information will be visible."

Numerous civil liberties organizations have argued that the law violates privacy rights. Yet in collusion with the Obama administration, Congress has refused to propose protecting personal privacy.

Quoted by the "New York Post," the physician appointed to establish the nation's electronic medical database, Doctor David Blumenthal, said that the system is designed to get doctors to bow to a higher authority by using "clinical decision support."

In essence, this means that—as stated by the "Post"—computers "will be telling doctors what to do." As a result, the newspaper said, some analysts predict that many physicians will protest the system, which would impose penalties on doctors who refrained from allowing computers to dictate treatments to administer.

Beware of the Obamacare Bureaucracy

As the law currently stands, Obamacare also will force taxpayers to submit their personal health information to the IRS. The tax mandate within the Act will open more opportunities for bureaucrats to destroy your privacy. From 2008 to 2011, several IRS workers were fired or charged for spying on personal information of celebrity taxpayers. The addition of mandatory health data when submitting IRS forms will give such hackers additional motivation to snoop, particularly into the lives of celebrities.

Allied with doctors or bureaucrats, your political enemies with insider access to bureaucrats or corrupt physicians will have instant access to your medical data. A column in "USA Today" described the process that was set to begin in mid-December of 2013 as the "largest consolidation of personal data in the history of the republic. If you think theft is a problem now, wait until Uncle Sam serves up critical information on 300 million American citizens on a platter."

The federal bureaucracy will balloon to seemingly unimaginable and hard-to-manage levels largely due to Obamacare, putting your personal info at risk of theft. The information that you're required to submit to the IRS will be shared and analyzed by the U.S. Department of Homeland Security and the Department of Justice—which all will receive your Social Security number as well.

The potential for abusing the personal data of individual Americans will become "staggering" as the critical information is stored in one central hub. "For one thing, the hub will have all the details needed to steal identities and fraudulently access credit," said Stephen T. Parente and Paul Howard in their "USA Today" column.

Squeezed by the urgency to meet extremely tight deadlines for implementing Obamacare in pre-designated phases, the administration has refused to specify what safeguards if any are being implemented to protect personal privacy. Journalists were finally able to discover the names of two vendors working to create the database after that info was inadvertently posted on the Web by a state insurance commissioner.

This bloated bureaucracy will give investigators and potentially thieves instant access to virtually all of your personal information. "This hub will achieve what has, until now, only appeared in pulp thrillers—a central database linking critical state and federal data on every U.S. citizen for real-time access," the Parente-Howard column said.

This vast crevasse in the information database is expected to open the doors to widespread fraud. As reported by the "New York Times," a 2012 report by the RAND Corporation predicts that the federal Medicare and Medicaid programs will lose up to $98 billion due to the resulting data leaks.

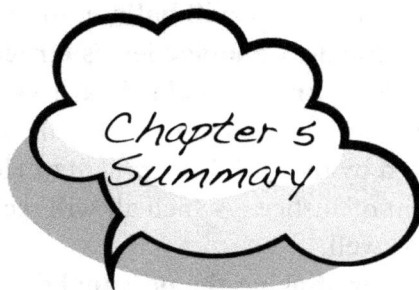

Chapter 5 Summary

Your personal privacy and the personal information of your entire family is about to be spread wide open for public view and potential identity theft. The Obama administration and the Democrat-controlled Senate have made no effort whatsoever to patch the upcoming privacy leaks.

6

Obamacare Provisions Will Sock People Nationwide

Theft: The U.S. government will "legally steal" or withhold the tax refund of any person who fails to obtain a health insurance policy deemed as qualified by bureaucrats.

Stupid rules: Your current employer will be required to ask you how much your spouse earns, even if you believe such queries are "none of their business."

Age discrimination: Blatantly discriminating against older citizens, the government will only allow people under age 30 to buy catastrophic health plans.

Obamacare Attacks All Levels of Society

People from virtually all professions and income levels will suffer economically and perhaps physically as a direct result of Obamacare's bureaucratic and senseless rules.

According to research by the Heritage Foundation, due to Obamacare at least half of people who have already been on Medicare "will no longer be able to keep the coverage they have."

Adding salt to the wounds of seniors, Obamacare will also make coverage for them more expensive due to new taxes imposed on the makers of drugs and health products.

Writing for the Foundation, Robert E. Moffitt, PhD, said that as a result of the Affordable Health Care Act the "solvency of the Medicare program will continue to weaken."

As a result, Moffitt said, the number of seniors covered by Medicaid will drop to one out of every eight people in that sector, down from the current one out of every four.

"With the retirement of 77 million baby boomers beginning in 2011, the Medicare program will have to absorb an unprecedented demand for medical services," Moffitt said. "For the next generation of senior citizens, finding a doctor will be more difficult and waiting times for doctor appointments are likely to be longer."

Obamacare Will Damage the Healthcare Industry

Doctor shortage: By 2025 after Obamacare kicks into full gear, the American population will have a projected 124,000 fewer doctors than needed, according to a report by the American Association of Medical Colleges.

Repair efforts: Doctor Moffitt states bluntly that "Obamacare has not ameliorated the growing problems of projected physician shortage and has surely made it worse."

Congressional tinkering: Congress had designed a Medicare physician payment update formula called the Sustainable Growth Rate. Yet due to the draconian nature of these pre-designated cutbacks, politicians who have no medical experience will keep making annual parliamentarian gyrations to ensure that this specific aspect of Congress' own destructive legislation never kicks into gear, according to a Heritage Foundation article by John O'Shea, M.D.

Higher taxes: During his first presidential campaign in 2008, Barack Obama promised never to increase taxes on the middle-class. However, the diverse hodge-podge of middle-class tax increases imposed upon Obamacare's enactment in 2010 will result in "lost wages and (lost) international competitiveness, while reducing families' wages just as surely as an income tax hike would," Curtis S. Dubay said in a Foundation article. Many analysts have agreed that Obamacare is the "largest single tax hike in human history."

Problems Intensified

According to a wide variety of government reports and analysis by various political commentators, Obamacare will result in a huge variety of other specific problems. Among them:

Penalties: Families earning less than $250,000 but with high-end health insurance policies will be forced to pay an "excise tax."

Separate funding: For the first time, hospital insurance payroll tax rate increases will fund a new entitlement separate from Medicare.

Slow economy: The high-tax, big-spending liberal legislation will slap a new Obamacare tax on investment income for couples earning more than $250,000 per year, ultimately slowing investments and dragging down the nation's economy. This reckless tax is designed to force wealthy people to pay for the health care of people such as drug addicts and criminals shot during robberies, and also to fund the federally mandated expansion of Medicaid.

Forced servitude: Taxpayers will be forced to pay the Obamacare tax whether they want to or not, the first time in American history that the government has required people to buy something.

Transition: After retiring or being booted out of office by voters in 2010 and 2012, many former Congressmen are no longer in office and thus no longer have to face the political consequences of the reckless healthcare legislation that they enacted.

Chapter 6
Summary

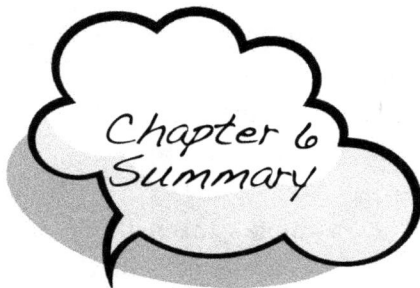

Virtually all Americans will suffer economically and perhaps physically as a result of Obamacare, even if they have previously supported or liked the legislation.

7
Mandatory Tax

Employment: The high prices mandated by Obamacare will prohibit lots of employers from giving entry-level jobs to many young people.

Low quality: The overall quality of healthcare is not guaranteed to improve, even for consumers who purchase higher-priced health insurance policies.

Disturbing reality: If Obamacare had never passed, more people would be retaining or getting employer-funded health insurance.

Runaway Federal Spending Accelerates

The most controversial aspect of Obamacare remains the requirement that taxpayers fund their own insurance in cases where employers do not supply such coverage and the person or family earns too much to qualify for Medicaid, or is covered by Medicare.

Critics call these "one-size-fits-all insurance plans." Even people with employer-funded policies face penalties if such plans fail to meet the federal government's rules.

In a show of arrogance by the federal government, only one individual—the secretary of the U.S. Department of Health and Human Services—will have the power to deem any particular insurance policy as meeting the required "essential benefits."

Behaving as if he is royalty with heavenly power, President Obama and his crony HHS secretary have made the controversial decision that all healthcare plans must pay for contraceptives. Amazingly, a future U.S. President could easily feel the opposite.

Sadly, as a result of this idiotic legislation over time the requirements imposed by Obamacare will be subject to the whims and political preferences of which politicians serve in the nation's highest-elected positions at any given time.

Adding to these concerns, during 2013 Americans with employer-funded health insurance had to wait for their bosses to make critical decisions.

Large, medium-size and even some small companies needed to decide whether to and how to obtain health insurance for their employees, or whether to drop such policies.

Obamacare Generated a Confusing Maze of Necessary Choices

Americans impacted by these critical choices also included children, young adults currently covered on their parents' policies, and adults covered on their spouses' employer-funded plans. Any person within those categories whose parents or spouse suddenly dies, or who gets an immediate divorce would face a critical chore of proving that they were insured or otherwise face steadily increasing federal penalties.

Behind-the-scenes chaos erupted through 2013 as employers, some frantic or confused, rushed to make critical decisions before the impending deadlines. In many cases these rules forced corporations to spend critical and expensive personnel hours working on these issues. These chores resulted in "soft" unlisted expenses that did not go directly to insurance companies. All along, whether they wanted to admit this or not, the firms essentially began "working for the government" in order to fulfill the requirements.

People will have to pay for coverage from "qualified plans" if their employers stop paying for their health insurance. Otherwise the individuals must enroll in Medicaid if qualifying as low-income or unemployed. The process that individuals ensure when purchasing their own policies will involve a complex maze of government-run Websites, or at state-operated offices similar to Department of Motor Vehicles facilities.

Consumers purchasing policies on their own via these bureaucratic government offices or Websites need to avoid getting fooled by the supposed quality of policies that are offered. For the most part citizens will be given a maze of options listed as platinum, gold, silver or bronze categories. Cnsumers need to know that the higher-priced policies will not necessarily result in better-quality health care. Buying a platinum-level policy should never be considered the equivalent of purchasing a top-of-the-line luxury automobile

Instead of offering varying steps of patient-care quality, the numerous plans at the platinum through bronze levels offer differing amounts of deductibles and co-pay fees. Consumers who choose to buy pricy gold- and platinum-level policies will end up with higher up-front premium payments than the silver and bronze levels. People choosing the higher-rung policies will pay lower co-pays and lower deductibles than consumers with bronze- and silver-level policies.

During 2013, people who have purchased their own health insurance needed to remain mindful that their policies might not eventually meet the government's arbitrary standard as a "qualified plan." There was no guarantee that a high-deductible plan would eventually meet the government's mandatory criteria. Thus, consumers who paid for their own policies needed to call their sales representatives or make direct inquiries to the firms to ensure that the criteria had been met.

Chapter 7
Summary

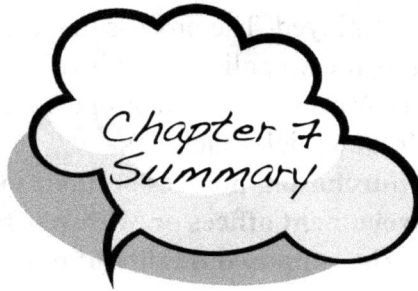

In many ways for average American citizens the reckless rules imposed by Obamacare will emerge as confusing—as difficult-to-understand as IRS forms. Americans need to understand these regulations, whether they want such policies or not. Otherwise consumers might end up paying excessive penalties to the Internal Revenue Service.

8
Expect Harsh Penalties For Violators

Penalties: After several years of increases in fine levels, annual penalties will reach up to a whopping $2,085 for any family that fails to purchase a "qualified plan."

Medicaid: People who buy their own standard policies will start paying more, the government's scheme to generate necessary funds for boosting Medicaid.

Young adults suffer: Many companies will stop or avoid funding health insurance for entry-level workers before those employees get dumped into Medicaid.

Beware of Excessive Fines

Obama's socialist bureaucrats and cronies are eager and ready to yank fine money from any taxpayer who dares avoid getting authorized health insurance policies.

These hassles begin as taxpayers submit their annual U.S. income tax forms to the IRS. The new rules require that filers attach a one-page document to their annual tax returns, similar to the way that taxpayers already had been doing yearly with their employer-provided W2 forms.

As of early 2013 the inept IRS bureaucrats in Washington, D.C., still had not yet released or shown the public actual copies of what this new form will look like.

Desperate for definitive answers that never came, numerous analysts and bloggers began distributing mock-up forms that they believed would look like the eventual documents.

Viewed on various unaffiliated Websites, most of these example forms look fairly identical—everything based on what observers know that Obamacare must require.

Most mock-up forms feature a maze of confusing boxes that would have to be filled out in order for taxpayers to meet stringent qualification processes set by the IRS.

The top third of these example forms feature at least 13 questions that taxpayers will be required to answer regarding their qualified policies. Under this, there is an "affordability" section where taxpayers must answer at least three questions about policy costs—all in direct relation to the amount of income listed within income filings.

An additional section would require that taxpayers list or acknowledge at least three types of exemptions that they might qualify for—answering "yes" or "no" in each of these categories.

Finally, at the bottom of the section on the page taxpayers would be required to check off each specific month of the calendar year that they were covered by a government-qualified plan. This would be necessary because Obamacare, working in collusion with the IRS, requires that each taxpayer have such a policy for at least ten months out of every calendar year.

Follow These Rules or Pay Big Fines

Although the form will be only one page long, the process likely will confuse many taxpayers due to the complexity of the required questions. People who fail to complete and submit this form properly face the possibility of steep fines. You can expect lots of frustrated taxpayers to become angry when the IRS withholds their refunds for either failing to submit the form or giving documentation that does not meet standards that the bureaucrats have set.

As of early 2013, the IRS still had failed to announce how long bureaucrats estimate that the form will take average taxpayers to fill out and to submit. Some observers fear that although only a single page the document will take several hours to complete due to its confusing maze of income levels and requirements.

Adding insult to injury, the IRS also has not announced how much the agency estimates that the form will cost taxpayers to have professional tax preparation firms to complete. In recent years the IRS has offered simple one-page EZ forms, often used by low-income taxpayers. Due to the new Obamacare provisions, the popular one-page process no longer will exist—replaced by a minimum two-page process.

Taxpayers used to completing their required annual returns on their own will essentially be "left in the dark" on whether they have properly completed and submitted the new forms. Some observers fear that this could tend to make at least some taxpayers feel more reliant on tax-preparation professionals, thereby adding a financial burden on such individuals.

The hassles of completing the required forms will increase multi-fold when taxpayers begin to realize the need to amass many types of additional forms. The days of submitting only financial information will be gone. Under the new system, taxpayers will have to amass necessary proof-of-insurance documentation. The amount of time needed to contact insurance providers in order to get the required forms also has not been calculated. In some instances taxpayers might not get the necessary data in time. Insurance companies also are busy familiarizing themselves with the process.

Companies that provide qualified insurance policies for their workers also will be required to send that information to

the IRS along with the standard W-2 data. This, in turn will also increase the amount of time and expense that American industries must expend in order to comply with Obamacare. Exactly how much of these costs might be passed on to consumers in the form of higher prices for products and services remains a matter of debate and extensive economic analysis.

Penalties Gradually Increase

Taxpayers who are uninsured for three or more months in any calendar year will be punished with fines or having their refunds withheld.

During the initial years of required forms starting in 2014, taxpayers will be fined one percent of their gross income or a $95 flat fee—whichever amount is higher. The percentage-of-income fines cap out at a maximum $295.

Starting in 2014 the annual flat-fee fine gradually gets higher through 2016, eventually topping out at $695 or a whopping 2.5 percent of the person's gross income (whichever is higher.)

Wretched provisions of Obamacare as passed by Congress enable the IRS to seize tax refunds from taxpayers who either fail to or refuse to pay the fines. In cases where fines remain outstanding but the taxpayer is not due a refund, the agency will be authorized to garnish the funds from bank accounts, freeze checking and savings accounts, garnish the individual's paychecks or slap liens onto the person's property.

Numerous individuals, groups or organizations do not need to comply with the mandate due to exemptions authorized by Congress. These include:
- People who entered the USA illegally
- Taxpayers who prove financial hardship yet fail to qualify for Medicaid
- People incarcerated in state penitentiaries or county jails

- Those already covered by federal health programs, such as American Indians
- People under age 30 who enroll in catastrophic insurance plans, as long as they can meet the requirements of plans deemed qualified by government bureaucrats
- People who are members of specific religious organizations
- People already enrolled in Medicare, Medicaid or other government health care programs

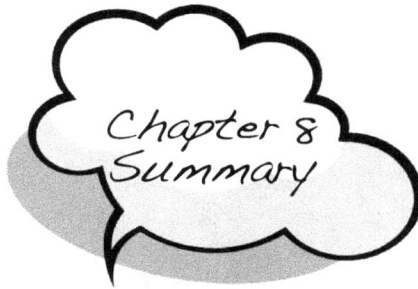

Chapter 8 Summary

American taxpayers will be saddled with new required IRS paperwork mandated by Obamacare. Those unable to figure out the forms likely will need to pay fees to tax-preparation professionals. Taxpayers also will need time to amass required documentation. Individuals and families that fail to or refuse to submit the paperwork in a manner that bureaucrats deem as appropriate will face fines that can include withholding tax refunds, garnishing wages, freezing bank accounts or property liens.

Eveything comes down to money. A doctor who refuses to follow the government's guidelines risk losing potential pay from insurance companies, Medicare or Medicaid.

9

Political Cronies Will Make Your Health Decisions

Cronies: Lacking medical education, cronies chosen by politicians will start making your critical health care decisions, passing those requirements on to doctors.

Outcasts: Your doctor must obey the bureaucrats' orders regarding your health care, or potentially face banishment from the medical profession

Power: You and your physicians will lack any power to protest the arbitrary and politically motivated decisions regarding your health care

Obey Bureaucrats or Suffer Severe Consequences

You can escape potential fines by legally and honestly submitting the required paperwork to the IRS and by purchasing an "authorized" insurance policy.

Even taxpayers who complete that phase, however, then must allow federal bureaucrats to control what your doctor can do regarding your medical care.

In essence, panels comprised of people who never attended medical school will be issuing directives on how and when doctors can treat you for specific medical conditions.

Thus, for the first time in history the federal government will begin dictating health care treatments for all Americans—while robbing doctors of the ability to make certain decisions regarding your treatment.

Everything comes down to money. A doctor who refuses to follow the government's guidelines risks losing potential pay from insurance companies, Medicare or Medicaid.

Kissing up to the high-power insurance industry, Congress approved the critical Section 1311 (H)(1) of the Act. That provision allows insurance firms to withhold payment to any doctor who fails to or refuses to adhere to the dictates of bureaucrats.

Is There No Way to Fight the Devil?

In essence, this new infrastructure is the equivalent to the notorious "star chamber," an English court of law in the Palace of Westminster prior to 1641. Many historians believe that body held court sessions in secret without requiring witnesses or indictments.

Many opponents of Obamacare insist that the draconian infrastructure of the USA's new health care Act similarly issues directives whether or not people want them.

One of the most powerful people in the world, even though never directly elected by the people, will become the person appointed by the president as the Secretary of Health and Human Services.

Under provisions of the Act, that person will have the power to implement government-imposed rules that he or she deems as necessary to improve the quality of health care—while also striving to slash the government's medical expenses.

Shockingly, this person is never required to have any medical training or experience whatsoever. These arbitrary, hit-and-miss powers will impact everything from the medical procedures performed by pediatric physicians to internists, oncologists and anesthesiologists.

Many critics worry that some rulings might tend to favor

certain healthcare professionals or specific manufacturers. Everything ultimately will hinge on politics rather than working in the best interests of consumers.

Political Cronies Will Rule Your Life

A federally appointed panel labeled with the bureaucratic name, the 15-member "Independent Payment Advisory Board," often called IPAB, will make many of these critical decisions regarding your personal healthcare.

Sadly, there is absolutely no requirement that these panelists have any medical training or experience. Instead of having the primary goal of giving you the best possible health care, the stated objective of these panelists will be to "cut costs."

When and if these panelists collectively make decisions that ruin the quality of healthcare or result in inefficiencies within the medical industry they will not have to face voters. Any senior citizens unhappy with the panel's actions will have no recourse, partly because the IPAB panel will work independently away from the general public.

To many people learning these startling details for the first time the mere set-up of the IPAB panel might seem like something from a science fiction film or horror movie.

Such perceptions become even more disturbing from the viewpoint of many consumers who receive additional facts about IPAB.

This panel's non-stop, primary job will be to locate and implement cuts to the vital health care services provided to seniors, everything from hospitals and hospices to physicians.

To say that IPAB "will cut benefits" would be misleading. However, the panel can work steadily to push down the amounts that the government pays for specific services, medicines or procedures—everything from cardiac surgeries to knee replacements.

Critics worry that while working diligently to cut costs the panel will eventually slash some government-mandated fee levels for specific treatments to excessively low levels. Some observers fear that when and if certain authorized fee levels plummet to critically low levels, service providers such as hospitals and doctors no longer would be able to provide specific treatments.

The President and Congress Can Claim "Plausible Deniability"

The Obamacare infrastructure is designed to cause long-term failures in the USA's medical industry, largely as a result of the IPAB setup.

Bureaucrats and politicians will become enraged upon reading or hearing the following fiery analysis. Yet there's no getting around the fact that by forming IPAB our congressmen and senators are exposing themselves as cowards.

Rather than standing tall and making medical expense cuts themselves, these idiotic elected leaders want a system where they can essentially "wash their hands of blame."

Thus, from the perspective of these elected leaders, the creation of IPAB serves as an excellent way for the politicians to avoid having to make extremely unpopular decisions.

Almost as if Mafia dons who order their gangsters to handle all the dirty work, Congress set up a system where IPAB formally "recommends" service or fee-level cutbacks. As required by the Act, each year the panel must submit its budget-, fee-, and service-cutting recommendations.

These recommendations automatically become effective, unless Congress decides to jump into the process and enacts different changes in Medicare that ultimately lead to the same level of savings. To the dismay of many critics, this means that IPAB will serve as a "lawmaking body," although never elected by the people.

James W. Forsythe, M.D., H.M.D.

Obamacare Supporters Label Opponents as "Biased"

Opponents of this draconian panel have emerged from both sides of the political aisle, including politicians who previously supported Obama's reckless health care act.

Thumbing their noses at the American people the politically demented nincompoops who first drafted the legislation in 2010 added a devilish provision.

Amazingly, as enacted by Congress in March 2010, the politicians essentially created a proverbial "doomsday clock."

Few people could deny that such an analysis is far off track. Everything comes down to the fact that following more than seven years of step-by-step additions to the Obamacare infrastructure, Congress would be allowed only a miniscule period of time during which the politicians could repeal the IPAB panel.

Taking a devilish step from the playbook of the 16th Century Italian politician Niccolò Machiavelli, Congress mandated that any proposal to repeal IPAB can only be submitted between January 1, 2017, and February 1, 2017. At least as dictated by Obamacare, no proposals to eliminate IPAB can be submitted before or after that time frame.

Multiplying this buffoonery, the pea-brained congressional politicians from Obama's first term also stipulated that any repeal of IPAB would have to occur no later than August 15, 2017.

All this idiocy is viewed as pure nonsense by some observers. They point out the fact that under the United States' republic form of government no specific body of Congress is allowed to dictate the actions or scheduled times of any future Congress.

Putting additional salt on the wounds suffered by American taxpayers and seniors as a result of Obamacare, many of the politicians approved the Act likely will be long gone by the time the primary infrastructure of the system reaches full force in 2017.

As authorized by the Constitution and various other federal laws, Obama's second and final term in the presidency will officially end in January 2017 on the heels of the 2016 presidential election. Thus, at the point where Obama leaves office, he no longer would have to face the potential wrath of voters angered by his health care Act or by the arbitrary and devilish nature of IPAB.

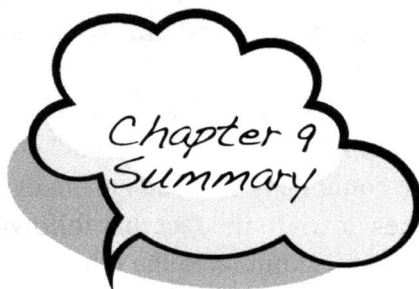

Chapter 9
Summary

Bureaucrats with absolutely no medical experience or education will make vital decisions regarding American health care, impacting everyone—especially seniors. The panel will not be held accountable to voters, although acting as a "lawmaking body." Lots of people appointed to this 15-member panel are likely to be political cronies.

10
Obamacare Will Attack Senior Citizens

Sudden raid: Despite claims to the contrary, Obamacare is raiding precious funds from the essential Medicare program vital to economically disadvantaged families

Weaken deductions: Until recently Americans paying federal taxes have been able to deduct medical expenses from their returns. Obamacare will reduce those advantages.

Hurting savers: Starting in 2013, the Obamacare system began limiting the amount of tax-free contributions that Americans can make to Flexible Savings Accounts.

Medicare Recipients Will Suffer

Some devious and unscrupulous politicians and bureaucrats have been trying to deceive the public. These ultra liberals want you to believe that plans to slash Medicare spending will keep that program solvent.

Quite to the contrary, however, politicians are robbing money from Medicare to help augment their Obamacare scheme. And, sadly, none of these purloined funds are being set aside to help keep Medicare strong for the future.

Instead, people under 65 years old who do not yet qualify for Medicare will benefit from these ripped-off funds that some critics say are being "robbed" from that program in order to finance Obamacare.

Desperate to shield the Act from criticism, some of its advocates have tried to cloud the issue into making seniors believe the purloined funds will help Medicare. However, the Director of the Congressional Budget Office and the chief actuary of Medicare have agreed that the money transfer will not extend the program's long-term life.

Understand the "Donut Hole"

The so-called "donut hole" in the Medicare program has caused financial hardship for many seniors. This term refers to a requirement that has forced seniors to pay up to 100 percent of drug expenses in cases where within any calendar year a person purchases from $2,800 and $6,400 in prescriptions.

Advocates of Obamacare note that the Act will essentially "close the donut hole." To accomplish this, money that the federal government takes from taxpayers and pharmaceutical company rebates sent to consumers will gradually cover over this gap.

Some analysts have said that the donut hole has caused extreme financial hardship to seniors who have fallen within that category. For the most part most medical expenses up to the $2,800 level have been covered by Medicare Part D.

Seniors Need to Become Wary of Obamacare

Little-known Obamacare provisions that effect seniors will also potentially endanger the long-term health of such patients.

As authorized by the Act, the new U.S. Preventative Services Task Force will work to reduce the preventative health care services for such patients.

The task force will work diligently to "increase" preventative services for Medicaid recipients, while also reducing preventative care services for seniors.

Controversy has already erupted as a result of these

paradoxical provisions. The panel sparked the public's ire by ruling that the government would no longer fund annual mammograms for women older than 74, or those ages 40 to 49.

Adding insult to injury, Obamacare actually encourages hospitals to spend as little as possible on seniors. Such institutions that prove they spend the least on such patients will get awarded bonus points under a system that began in October 2012.

At least from the perspective of opponents to Obamacare, a primary worry here is that hospitals will benefit by giving seniors the lowest-cost treatments possible, potentially the least effective. The potential danger that seniors will face heightens when taking into account the fact that the government will slap demerits on the hospitals that spend more on such patients.

Essentially, due to various provisions within the new law, hospitals across the United States will be aggressively competing with each other to give seniors the "most impersonal, lowest-cost, least effective care possible." Many seniors who have worked their entire adult lives to achieve at least some degree of dignity will find themselves treated like lower-class citizens.

Hospitals will increase their chances of avoiding demerits if they essentially "get rid" of patients and never see those individuals again after providing such basic services as knee or hip replacements. Hospitals that provide physical therapy for such patients within 30 days after those individuals are discharged will face demerits.

This dilemma sparks additional concern when taking into account the undeniable fact that studies have consistently shown that on average seniors survive longer within hospitals that spend more on their care.

Critical Questions Lead to Startling Answers

Doctors will receive more compensation for treating all non-elderly patients including Medicaid recipients than when

caring for seniors. Elderly people have a right to consider this offensive. Studies have consistently shown that seniors who consistently and regularly receive medical care live healthier and longer lives.

The cuts in the quality of health care for seniors will come as massive amounts of people reach age 65, the age when people qualify for Medicare. While supposedly caring for the needs of seniors, the government is actually showing disrespect for such individuals who for their whole lives have counted on eventually benefiting from the program.

Medicare will be spending $1,431 less per year on seniors in 2019 than the service would have expended had the new law never been enacted. This estimate was listed in a report entitled "National Health Expenditure Projections," published by "Health Affairs" in October 2010.

Some observers argue that the Medicare cuts will total $716 billion, while other critics claim the cuts will be "only" $575 billion. Each of these amounts is correct. The higher total marks the combined cuts beginning in 2010, while the lower total results from when cuts began in 2012.

In coming years as a result of the new law seniors will have an extremely difficult time getting basic medical procedures that had drastically improved the lives of many elderly people in recent decades. The Act's penalty and reward system will cut down on the access that seniors have to treatments that have helped prevent many elderly people from languishing in nursing homes or from remaining confined to wheelchairs. Some of these basic transformational services have included cataract operations, bypass surgery, knee replacements, angioplasty and hip replacements.

Doctors will earn substantially more for patients other than seniors. Some observers fear that as a result of these decreases in fee schedules seniors will have an extremely difficult time finding qualified physicians. The lower pay when treating such individuals will motivate doctors to seek other patients for such procedures as hip replacements. These are critical factors because numerous studies show that such treatments as knee replacements can save lives or at least increase a patient's life expectancy.

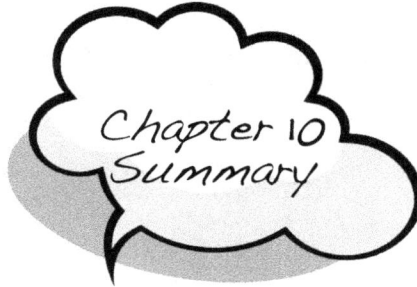

Chapter 10 Summary

If left unchanged, the Affordable Health Care Act will steadily and gradually erode the quality and amount of medical services provided to seniors by Medicare. Seniors will experience increased difficulty obtaining basic medical treatments shown to improve the overall health and quality of life of the elderly. Seniors lucky enough to schedule such services also will have to wait longer, perhaps even many months or even years. Doctors will become increasingly reluctant to treat seniors for serious illnesses, as federal panels strive to lower the amounts that Medicare pays doctors for treating the elderly.

The authors of Obamacare "spiced up" or sweetended the dregulations in a misguided effort to fool the public into believeing that the Act's benefits would autweigh the insurance-purchasing rule.

60

11

The Much-Hated Individual Mandate

Public opinion: Regular surveys of public opinion have consistently indicated that the public overwhelming dislikes being forced to purchase health care insurance.

Affordability: Many taxpayers, perhaps millions of them, will end up buying health care insurance policies but never be able to afford paying the deductibles.

Confusion: The inept and inefficient federal government has never issued an official publication on how employers and consumers should use Obamacare.

Government Incompetence

Behind-the-scenes political skullduggery prompted Congress to enact Obamacare's controversial mandate that requires taxpayers to purchase health care insurance policies.

High-paid lobbyists for the health insurance industry worked in the best interests of their employers in helping Congress to craft the legislation.

Desperate to protect their own business interests as well, pharmaceutical companies, health product manufacturers and some hospitals also helped with the legislation.

These political insiders who crafted Obamacare legislation agreed overall that the only way for the legislation to succeed was to force "invincibles" to purchase health care insurance. These are people ages 18 to 35 that have as an overall group a far less need for healthcare than others from the overall population.

Invincibles have a far lower death rate than other adults. The most prevalent cause of death or disability among invincibles are accidents such as car wrecks, extreme sports injuries, suicide or having unprotected sex with people who suffer from sexually transmitted diseases such as AIDS.

The crafters of Obamacare calculated that the proposed legislation would work only if the generally healthy "invincibles" were forced to acquire such policies. This way the invincibles would be forced to pay for the health coverage of older individuals and the similar expenses of people suffering from pre-existing medical conditions.

With their own best interests in mind, rather than the needs of the overall general public, through the actions of its lobbyists the health insurance industry made the "individual mandate" a strict requirement within the legislation.

Corruption Led to a Reckless Rush to Pass the Act

When quickly and haphazardly crafting the legislation, the self-serving lobbyists and the inept politicians whipped up the 2,500 pages of legislation without taking time for critical analysis. This was done during a 14-month period from January 2009, the month of Obama's first-term inauguration, through March 2010 when Congress narrowly approved the bill.

Callous, heartless and striving to serve only their warped political ideologies, many members of the House—particularly Democrats—had strived to ram the bill through Congress without even bothering to review the legislation. Congresswoman Nancy Pelosi, a San Francisco Democrat and the House Majority Leader at the time, had famously said that Congress needed to first pass the bill so that the politicians could "find out what's in it."

When first proposing and developing the legislation, the

politicians had what many observers might consider as the admirable goal of drastically slashing the number of uninsured Americans.

The number of uninsured U.S. citizens in 2010 had ballooned to an estimated 50 million people, up a whopping 32 percent from 38 million Americans in 2000. The problem got so bad that about one out of every five working-age citizens were uninsured.

However, many politicians went overboard on the legislation. Rather than merely striving to provide medical services to uninsured people, the corrupt, inept or incompetent lawmakers shifted some of the emphasis on Medicaid.

The U.S. Supreme Court Made a Political Decision

The overall issue and the potential to efficiently analyze the effort got clouded by the U.S. Supreme Court ruling that cleared the way for Obamacare. Technically, when considering any case or legal dispute, the court must rule on issues as a matter of law rather than for political reasons. However, when issuing their Obamacare ruling in 2012 the jurists overstepped their bounds by making a political choice, rather than basing their decision purely on legalities, some critics say.

Among the key issues here centers on the fact that states would be able to opt-out of the court's ruling that allowed for the expansion of Medicaid.

By early 2013 only a handful of states had announced that they had decided not to participate in Medicaid's poorly planned expansion as mandated by Obamacare. As a result, analysts admitted that they could not fully or accurately calculate what impact the legislation would have on Medicaid and ultimately on people that the legislation is designed to serve.

Any thorough analysis of long- and short-term advantages and disadvantages became almost impossible. Until that critical juncture officials had based their calculations on an original

Congressional Budget Office calculation that incorrectly assumed every state would be forced to participate.

Several years before that critical point, the self-serving political cronies and one-sided political lobbyists who crafted Obamacare needed to determine why many Americans had intentionally avoided buying such policies.

To almost no one's surprise, researchers focused on two primary factors. First, analysts found that many people without health insurance considered such purchases as a "waste of time and money." A huge percentage of people who thought this way were the healthy young "invincibles," who refused to face the fact that an accident or unexpected catastrophic illness could suddenly wipe out their finances.

Secondly, a huge number of Americans without health insurance policies viewed such plans as necessary and something that they wanted. But many of these individuals did not have such policies because: they could not afford to purchase them; they were already covered under employer-funded programs, or they failed to qualify for Medicaid.

The Massachusetts Health Care Model

When finalizing their ultimate Obamacare strategy in early 2010, the political cronies and lobbyists used as a model what then was the 3-year-old state-run Massachusetts mandatory health care insurance program.

There have never been any formal allegations or insulations that those who developed the eventual federal plan were corrupt. Even so, amid their shenanigans these characters must have realized that unless a purchase-insurance requirement or "mandate" were imposed, many Americans still would have refused to buy health care insurance—even if offered for extremely low fees.

Until the Bay State's program numerous individual states had tried unsuccessfully to launch health care programs. Those other states all had given citizens a right to refrain from making such purchases. Massachusetts changed the overall playing field by requiring its residents to purchase such plans.

By the time they started crafting Obamacare, the federal politicians, bureaucrats and lobbyists considered that liberal New England's state's plan a resounding success. Some participants claimed up to 97 percent of Massachusetts residents complied.

These co-conspirators on the federal level realized that the only way for the Act to work would be to "stick it to" taxpayers, making compliance mandatory. Subsequently, making a political rather than a judicial decision, the U.S. Supreme Court in 2012 ruled that Obamacare was a "tax" that Congress had the power to enact.

Obamacare Equals Runaway Government Spending

From the perspective of citizens opposed to huge runaway government, Obamacare became a literal nightmare come true even before the Act began to take full effect.

Opponents claimed that by taking away the will of the people and forcing United States citizens to buy something, politicians and the government had overstepped their bounds. Allegations of a "nanny state" began to flare.

Those who championed and supported Obamacare took a drastically opposing view. These individuals perceive the Act as the government's way of caring for people who are unwilling to or incapable of properly caring for themselves.

Proponents continue to claim that the "mandatory" provisions of Obamacare generate a long list of benefits for society as a whole. Perhaps most important, at least from the view of many who support the new law, insurance companies no longer will be able to deny coverage to patients who already have suffered from pre-existing health problems. Just as important, at least from their view, Obamacare prohibits insurance companies from placing caps on the amount of combined long-term benefits that people with pre-existing conditions can receive. This only could have become possible by forcing everyone to buy insurance. Essentially, as stated earlier, healthy people were forced to start paying for the care of sick individuals.

Some conservatives, Republicans, Libertarians and non-partisans—occasionally joined by steadily growing numbers of liberals—started complaining that Obamacare had evolved into full-scale socialism. Heated bickering erupted between the political right and left as to whether the new rules would hurt or help health care overall, or even potentially wreck the economy.

Opponents began claiming essentially that "we're going to fall down the same socialist and economic rat-hole that has engulfed Greece—and which is already steadily ravaging the rest of Europe." Under this line of thinking, the entire U.S. economy eventually would crumble largely as a result of Obamacare. Some opponents feared the damage would become so severe that U.S. taxpayers eventually might have to spend more than half of their incomes to support the massive, uncontrollable and runaway Big Government that Obamacare requires.

The Act's opponents feared that such developments eventually would lead to conditions where business and industry lose all motivation to develop new technologies, prompting Corporate America to avoid forming new ventures that might eventually prosper.

Essentially, from the perspective of those who despised Obamacare, the new regulations were tantamount to intentionally shooting yourself in the head—before using a tiny bandage in hopes of fixing the wound. Rather than helping, the bandage would fail to hold back the insurmountable loss of essential life-giving fluids.

Obamacare Supporters Applaud the Regulations

Refusing to accept any criticisms whatsoever, those who

continued to support Obamacare described the new rules as "the best solutions available."

To their way of thinking, society is far better off when government takes decisive actions to help the poor or people too ill to afford adequate health care. These advocates insist that the mandate is the "just, good and right" thing, essentially mirroring the "golden rule" taught by loving religions—to "do unto others as you would do unto yourself."

While such goals might sound admirable at face value, the Obamacare opponents refuse to embrace such deceptive and naïve rhetoric.

These opponents of the new law, many from the Republican, Libertarian, non-partisan and "Tea Party" political ideologies, have insisted that all socialist and communist societies are "corrupt and inefficient," no matter how well-intended such systems might seem.

The argument intensified even further when the liberals or Democrats complained that the demonic forms of capitalism that the U.S. government has always supported "took advantage of the little guy—feasting upon the middle-class and poor as if little field mice being slowly pecked upon by giant indiscriminate hawks."

Largely as a result of this crevasse generated by diametrically opposing viewpoints, Americans on both sides of the political and economic spectrum became more hotly divided than ever. Especially from 2011 well into 2013, a deeply divided Congress became bogged down in persistent gridlock on critical financial legislation.

Federal Employees Issued a Critical Warning

Liberals, conservatives and non-partisans all need to face a grim reality. No matter what political leanings each of us has, we all must realize and acknowledge the irrefutable statements made by the non-partisan Congressional Budget Office and by numerous highly experienced economists. Among their conclusions:

Cost overruns: Obamacare will balloon in costs to the federal government, far past the point that politicians and analysts had originally projected.

Lower services: As previously stated, largely as a result of these insufficient funds, coupled with the government's intentional strategy of slashing costs, the overall quality of services will continue to plummet.

Doctor shortages: Authorities from various federal and private organizations have already projected that by the 2015 to 2018 period, the U.S. will have more than 50,000 fewer medical doctors than needed. Those totals are expected to balloon significantly higher by 2025 and beyond.

Failures elsewhere: At least according to some observers, virtually all socialized medical care programs in other countries have failed miserably. Some of the worst examples are in Canada. Many of that nation's residents have been coming to the United States in order to get decent medical care, rather than wait many years in their own country for basic services. England is among numerous socialized-medicine countries where patients have been known to languish in hospitals without receiving adequate care.

Labor problems: The many flaws of Obamacare will essentially begin "feeding upon themselves." Among the worst provisions are stipulations that reward hospitals that spend the least on senior patients. Partly as a result, major medical corporations including firms that own and operate hospitals will start slashing staff levels or drastically cutting the pay of essential workers such as nurses. These situations, in turn, could result in labor strikes, such as those that already began in various U.S. communities in 2011, 2012 and 2013.

Convoluted Issues Abound

Due to the complexity of these issues, the "average American" seems to lack any grasp of the many issues that Obamacare will impose.

Many observers also wonder how President Obama's administration was able to push the Act through Congress after a short 14 months in office. This compared with former President Bill Clinton whose two-term administration failed to come close to getting any federal health care legislation proposed from January 1993 to January 2001.

Clinton's supposed failure in this regard, and Obama's ultimate "success" hinged on the unscrupulous mandate forcing the public to buy policies. During the 1990s, the insurance industry refused to back Clinton's efforts, which lacked a mandate provision. Obamacare placated the corporations' concerns by making the policies mandatory.

Sadly, however, when striking its deal with the Obama administration and with congressional Democrats, the health insurance industry refrained from making any promises on how much consumers would have to pay for policies.

The shocking result will increasingly force the supporters of Obamacare to acknowledge the fact that even before being enacted the law has resulted in:

Co-pay: Increases in the amounts that legitimate policy holders must pay to visit a physician or medical facility.

Deductibles: Ramping up for Obamacare to reach its full-growth in 2017 and beyond, in 2011 insurance companies started raising the total amounts that policyholders were required to pay out of their own pockets for annual medical care.

Premiums: Dismayed and angry policyholders started receiving annual letters stating that their monthly premiums had been raised. Essentially these consumers were being required to pay more for the same policies, without being given any specific reason for why or how these increases had occurred. This trend, in turn, made planning annual family budgets extremely difficult. Ultimately, well before going into full force Obamacare had already started chipping away at the spending power of American families.

Bureaucrats Tried to "Sweeten" the Deal

The authors of Obamacare "spiced up" or sweetened the regulations in a misguided effort to fool the public into believing that the Act's benefits would outweigh the insurance-purchasing rule. Among these deceptive tactics:

Help: Voters were told that Obamacare would give low-income people financial help in obtaining health insurance policies.

Bureaucracy grows: Americans were promised that the government assistance would come in the form of policy subsidies to qualified low-income individuals or families via exchanges or from Medicaid serving needy families.

Bargain prices: Obamacare supporters promised that low-income people could select from policies far below the regular market value, or even get coverage for "free."

Smoke and mirrors: Tax credits were promised to small business that decided to offer employee-funded insurance policies to their workers.

Medicaid balloons: Under the plan as originally envisioned and approved, the availability of Medicaid would be thrown wide open to millions of people who previously would never have qualified. As of 2010, the year Congress approved the Act, individuals or four-person families that earned less than $29,327 yearly in most states would qualify.

More Cloudy Issues Emerged

The U.S. Supreme Court put a proverbial fly in the ointment when ruling that the sweetening of Medicaid was unconstitutional, used as a coercive method of forcing Americans to purchase health insurance policies. Confusion resulted partly because the court also approved Obamacare and its "buy-insurance" requirement.

These paradoxical rulings muddied an already cloudy situation. Even before the court ruled, numerous states already had signaled their reluctance to participate in the ballooning of Medicaid. The controversy got even stickier when the original Obamacare law threatened to remove federal financial support to any state that refused to participate.

Such penalties if imposed upon any individual state would have extreme financial hardship on that jurisdiction.

Steeped in unnecessary bureaucracy and required paperwork, the confusion intensified when the court ruled that states could maintain current enrollment levels—rather than opening up the floodgates to streams of new recipients.

The importance of this dilemma comes into clear focus when considering the financial problems that states faced prior to Obamacare. Even before the Act's ill-advised passage in 2010 the exorbitant costs had forced many states to accept only the minimum number of Medicaid recipients.

This disturbing factor emerged as the primary reason why 26 states had filed separate lawsuits on this issue between when Obamacare became law in 2010 and when the court ruled in mid-2012. The states had cited the 14th Amendment to the U.S. Constitution, which would give them sovereignty from federal regulations.

In its controversial ruling that cleared the way for Obamacare, the court ruled in favor of those states opposing the Medicaid-growth requirement. Yet this development left states with the challenging choices of whether to maintain enrollment levels in

Medicaid. Any state that chooses to expand enrollment could qualify for what Obamacare advocates hailed as fantastic federal subsidies.

Prior to the passage of Obamacare, the federal government had covered an average of 57 percent of what each state pays toward Medicaid costs within its borders. All that instantly changed with the new law. When accepting "new eligibles," only those states that agree to participate through 2020 in Medicaid's enrollment expansions would have about 93 percent of those costs covered.

Our Government Flew the "Skull and Crossbones" Flag

Supporters of the Affordable Health Care Act argue that the 93-percent federal subsidies provide great incentive for states to participate, a significant jump from the 57-percent level of federal funds for pre-Obamacare enrollees in Medicaid.

By early 2013, Obamacare supporters and their profit-hungry insurance industry allies were hoping that the opposition of individual states would fade. Some observers hoped that the promise of larger hunks of the federal money pie would soften the objections. Among critical factors that observers began to track:

Potential growth: The number of uninsured people nationwide would decrease by 15 million by 2019, at least according to projections by some bureaucrats. Others disputed those calculations, fearing that the number of uninsured people would rise.

Added enticements: Rather than funneling funds only to Medicaid, the federal government also plans to pump money into the health insurance exchanges maintained by states. This complex formula earmarked for exchanges would be based on the income of each person or family acquiring policies, coupled with the levels of income that would enable a taxpayer to qualify for federal subsidies. The specific federal subsidies applied to an individual's or a family's insurance policy costs would hinge on a sliding scale, tracking whether a person's income increases or falls in comparison to the federal poverty level.

Sudden growth: The bureaucracy will surge in scope, breadth and power as the mandate clicks into full gear in 2014. Right when Medicare balloons in size, the exchanges will help subsidize the insurance coverage for people unable to qualify for that assistance. Obamacare proponents hope this giant, confusing and hard-to-navigate maze of bureaucracy will help many people who never previously had health insurance coverage, perhaps tens of millions of them.

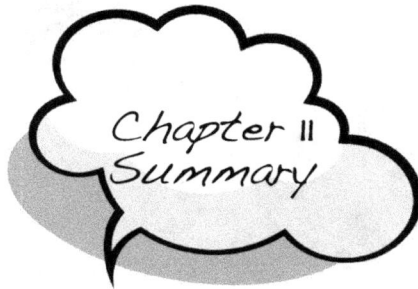

Chapter II Summary

The Medicaid expansion and subsidized exchanges will make the acquisition of health insurance policies extremely difficult for all Americans. As streams of doctors retire or intentionally leave the profession, a nationwide shortage of physicians will steadily surge to disturbing levels. These problems will in turn lower the quality of health care that Americans receive, as confused Americans scramble to purchase required policies or strive to determine if they qualify for Medicaid. Worsening matters from the perspective of many consumers and health care professionals, the continued reluctance of many states to participate in the Medicaid expansion will likely increase the confusion.

The cold, hard facts clearly point to the fact that the overall quality of Medicaid will decrease. The sudden surge of participants will force states to cut back in services.

12
Qualifying for Government Assistance

Confusion: The average American will never read voluminous books in order to determine where and how to qualify for government assistance on Obamacare.

Struggling families: The Affordable Health Care Act does nothing to give financial assistance to struggling middle-class families striving to comply with the mandate.

Growing funds: People lucky enough to have jobs will actually end up paying more out-of-pocket expenses in order to comply with Obamacare.

Tax increase: Now with the blessing of the U.S. Supreme Court, Obamacare is essentially the largest single tax increase in world history. The funds that individuals and families must spend to acquire health insurance policies are considered a "tax."

Where You Live Will Make a Huge Difference

Anyone seeking to participate in Medicaid for the first time, or who wants to receive financial help from the federal government in exchanges needs to know that "not everyone is equal" under Obamacare. Everything hinges on the state where a person lives

A person in one state might find himself blocked from potential participation in Medicaid because their jurisdictions refuse to expand. Meantime, that same individual might have qualified in a neighboring state that participates in Medicaid's growth.

Just as disturbing, some consumers are likely to discover that the rates offered on their own state exchanges are exorbitantly high, compared to levels posted on the government-operated Websites of neighboring states.

Potentially worsening matters to levels of great concern, residents of some low-populated states might find that only a handful of insurance companies compete for their business on the exchanges. This in turn could push up policy rates to excessive levels in such states, far above the fees charged to people in high-population states where insurance companies are projected to aggressively compete for business.

A state exchange will only give financial assistance to families with less than five people, but only if their total income is less than a specified multiple of the federal poverty line for such a group. As of 2010, that level for a four-person family was $88,200. The poverty-line total is likely to change yearly, thus adding more to the confusion involving Obamacare.

Families and individuals whose annual incomes are above the poverty line will still be able to buy policies, but not with federal financial help.

Proponents of Obamacare insist that consumers will benefit even if they earn more than the poverty level; the Act's supporters claim that health insurance policy rates will decrease.

But many opponents of the Act say otherwise. Lots of people who dislike Obamacare cite statistics showing that insurance rates already were shooting upward in 2012 and 2013, well in advance of the Act's full effects.

Expect Heavy Penalties for Violators

The government will harass, track down and heavily penalize all taxpayers who earn greater than the "maximum multiples" of poverty-line incomes, but who still fail to buy health insurance or enter Medicaid. Also, low-income people who either fail to or refuse to get coverage will face penalties.

The wage garnishments, the withholding of tax refunds and the issuance of tax liens, all mentioned earlier, are only a small portion of the "big brother" mentality.

Besides writing threatening letters to alleged violators, the bureaucrats might also threaten jail time although the statue lacks any criminal penalties. Quite understandably many people have a tremendous fear of the IRS.

Nonetheless, those who support the new law insist that only an extremely small percentage of taxpayers will have anything to fear. By some estimates more than 18 out of every 20 adults in the United States already have some form of health insurance.

Observers on both sides of this hot issue give diverging information. Proponents say that Medicaid's expansion will enable 14 million Americans to enter that program without having to pay anything out of their own pockets. Opponents insist that the Act will raise health care costs for all companies and individuals that purchase policies, while also increasing the number of uninsured.

Even if both sides are only partly correct a huge overall societal change is underway. The vast majority of people above the poverty line will have to pay, in many cases for the first time— while lower-income individuals pay little or nothing.

Penalize Successful People

Those who suffer the most financially as Obamacare initially clicks into full gear will be:

Medicaid: Taxpayers who earn too much to qualify for Medicaid, and

Subsidies: People whose incomes are too high for them to qualify for government subsidies when purchasing policies via the government-operated exchanges.

Understandably and for very good reasons, lots of the individuals who will be forced to purchase health insurance policies feel angry and frustrated.

The requirement forcing them to "buy something that they don't want" is a resounding slap in the face to many hard-working Americans. Many of them grew up being taught that we live in a free-market society where every person has a right to choose or to avoid any product or service.

The various escape clauses mentioned earlier, for everyone from prisoners to illegal immigrants, only heightens the frustration among some law-abiding citizens. Those who struggle to earn good incomes while obeying the laws will be forced to pay for the medical services of illegal aliens who have never paid a penny to the U.S. government.

Many of today's middle-aged taxpayers and seniors had to work hard to purchase or to qualify for health insurance when they were young adults. Conversely, under the new law many people under age 27 will be able to sidestep the mandate by remaining on their parents' health insurance policies.

Even people praising Obamacare need to acknowledge a flaw in this sector. Remember, as previously stated young adults are the "invincible" individuals that Obamacare needs in order to work with efficiency, since those individuals are far less likely to become catastrophically ill than the rest of the general population.

Medicaid's Runaway Growth Becomes Critical

Another serious flaw within Obamacare grows from its over-reliance on the expansion of Medicaid, which has been a terribly flawed and inefficient bureaucracy. Loaded with excessive wasteful inefficiencies, Medicaid was first enacted in 1965 during the first year of former President Lyndon Johnson's single four-year term.

From the view of many people, Medicaid started with the noteworthy objective of providing health coverage for the poorest families. Since its inception, Medicaid's costs have been covered by states and the federal government.

The amount and breadth of inefficiencies steadily grew, as states got stuck with running Medicaid's daily operations. The federal government became the bossy, know-it-all big brother, determining enrollment qualifications and operational procedures.

Initially, families with pregnant women or children under age seven emerged as the biggest recipients. People with children ages 7 to 18 fell in the next-highest percentage of Medicaid enrollees, followed by the elderly or disabled and working parents.

Inefficiency Increased as Medicaid Grew

The inefficiencies within Medicaid increased multi-fold when the government gave individual states the option to enroll more people—past the levels at which the feds had agreed to provide matching funds. Thus states had to cover the costs of adding such individuals.

A provision within Obamacare to allow childless adults to receive Medicaid coverage emerged as a key issue in motivating states to file lawsuits against the Act.

Right on target, even after the eventual Supreme Court ruling, some politicians and particularly Republicans had labeled the expansion of Medicaid as the federal government's way of inflicting extortion upon the states.

Streams of critics pointed out that via the Act as initially approved the federal government had been bullying states. At the time of its enactment, the new law threatened to withhold funds from any state that refused to or failed to expand its Medicaid program in ways that the federal government demanded.

In the wake of the Supreme Court's ruling, the governors of several states including Rick Perry of Texas voiced their strong opinions that the inept federal government had spawned numerous weaknesses and deficiencies in Medicaid.

Hitting the proverbial bull's-eye dead center, numerous politicians including Perry equated the expansion of Medicaid to essentially trying to put an additional 1,000 passengers on the ill-fated Titanic right before it sank in 1912 in the North Atlantic.

Steeped in political double-talk and striving to spin the issue to their advantage, over-the-top big-spending liberals insisted that despite such descriptive comparisons that Medicaid likely would continue to thrive. These pro-Obamacare advocates continue to spew analysis that would boggle the minds of many Republicans, Libertarians or Tea Party supporters.

Believing their own hogwash, the supporters of Obamacare seem to conclude that the U.S. government is some sort of bottomless pit with endless financial resources.

Snubbing their noses at American taxpayers, even as the federal budget deficit skyrocketed past $16 trillion in 2012, Obamacare supporters insist that all federal entitlement programs such as Social Security can efficiently continue to grow. These individuals insist that the largest federal entitlement programs can and should expand unabated over time while raking in ever-increasing revenues from taxpayers.

Federal Bureaucrats Disagree With the Liberal Assertions

Claims of Obamacare's long-term efficiency and that entitlement programs can continue growing without letup are contrary to the assertions of federal financial experts who work to study the U.S. government's current and projected finances.

Various reports issued by the non-partisan Congressional Budget Office in 2011 and 2012 state unequivocally that Social Security would go bust within 20 years. From the perspective of these analysts federal entitlement programs are tantamount to legalized Ponzi schemes that eventually will go bust.

However, under the way of thinking embraced by Obamacare advocates, the all powerful and mighty federal government will do everything in its power to prevent Medicare, Medicaid, Social Security and all other entitlement programs from sinking.

Some might view this as a resounding slap directly in the face of common sense. The USA's federal credit rating has steadily been downgraded since the international financial crisis of 2008. With the federal government spending far more money yearly than it receives in revenues, the so-called "dead-end" could be just around the corner for entitlement programs and for the entire U.S. economy.

When and if that happens, the locomotive that operates in the form of the U.S. "gross national product" or GNP eventually could plummet off a fiscal cliff.

This same scenario already has happened in recent years in such diverse nations as Greece and Spain, where entire economies have been ravaged. With this in mind, the notion of proceeding as if "all entitlements will be okay if left untouched," is reckless and highly dangerous for both the current economy but also for future generations.

Medicaid's Overall Quality Will Decrease

The cold, hard facts clearly point to the fact that the overall quality of Medicaid will decrease. The sudden surge of participants will force states to cut back in services that they offer through the program.

As of the time this book was published more than 40 states had agreed to expand their Medicaid services. A handful of states were able to opt-out of the expansion without incurring any financial fines, thanks to the Supreme Court's 2012 ruling.

The federal government will cover the bulk of Medicaid benefits received by its participants. Uncle Sam promises that states will only pay a small percentage.

States that benefit the most will be in low-income regions like Alabama. Those regions have more people per-capita below the federal poverty line than the average per-state nationwide. Many people of low income will get Medicaid for the first time, particularly in impoverished states.

Much of this surge in Medicaid participants will occur because from 2014 through 2017 the federal government will cover all costs of newly eligible people in the program. The federal payment levels will steadily decrease to 90 percent of total costs by 2020.

Many state-level politicians insist they will not be fooled by this up-front sweetener. Lawmakers from high-population states like Florida call Medicaid's expansion a "tragedy in the making." They worry that federal participation might drop significantly after 2020.

Many Will Learn of Medicaid for the First Time

More concern emerges when factoring in the fact that people who previously would have qualified for Medicaid but never joined will enter the program for the first time. Until now lots of these people never knew they could join or they lacked motivation.

This is where the states should expect to get walloped. Some needy people who could have qualified in the past for Medicaid had never tried to sign up into that program before. When these previously qualified individuals sign up after Obamacare starts, a state will only get paid by the federal government at the 57-percent level—the same rate that had been set for those individuals prior to Obamacare.

Some analysts including writers for the "New England Journal of Medicine" have expressed concern. They worry that previously qualified new enrollees will devastate the budgets of state governments.

By some estimates immediately prior to Obamacare only an average of 62 percent of people who had previously been qualified to join Medicaid signed up for that program. The percentage was lower in some high-population states like Florida and Texas. Those states ranked in the 44 percent to 48 percent range.

Other high-population states quickly rushed in to expand their Medicaid participation. The California state government jumped on board. Golden State officials estimated that the number of people participating in Medicaid would surge there by a half million.

Nonetheless, states will eventually need to work hard to limit Medicaid service and to slash costs, according to an analysis by the Heritage Foundation. Some bureaucrats hope that the federal government's subsidy payments offered via the exchanges will help offset this dilemma.

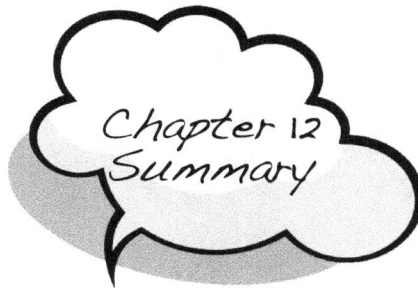

Chapter 12 Summary

The expansion of Medicaid likely will create a severe financial burden on individual states. Over time those jurisdictions will have to cut back on Medicaid services, limiting fees for covering certain medical checkups or treatments. Although many people will get medical coverage for the first time via Medicaid its quality will decrease.

The Act's detrimental provisions impacting small businesses could generate a negative and irreversible "whirlpool effect" due to the countless destructive factors hidden within Obamacare.

13
Impacts on Small Businesses

Small business nationwide and many of their employees will suffer extreme hardships as a direct result of Obamacare.

Crafters of the Act added numerous incentives designed to motivate small businesses to provide health insurance coverage. Yet the exorbitant costs will actually lower the amount of such participation.

Employees likely will suffer the brunt of these changes. Many workers will be forced to scramble to buy their own health insurance when their employers drop plans.

Other negative impacts will slam part-time workers in cases where companies drop or choose not to pursue coverage for such workers. These problems likely will get compounded when small businesses transform full-time jobs into part-time positions, in some instances the only way for such ventures to comply with the Act's new provisions.

The slap against small business will pose a serious threat to the fragile American economy. Economists say that such ventures serve as the backbone of the current and future prosperity of the United States.

Small Businesses Face of Maze of Options

Obamacare sets a sliding scale upon which small businesses can benefit via tax credits. The potential benefits to each business depend on its size, employee levels and the amount of coverage that the venture provides to employees.

This is different from the health insurance exchanges where individual taxpayers can seek to have their policy expenses partially subsidized by the federal government, and from Medicaid that pays all medical expenses of participants.

The tax credits system designed to assist small businesses likely will put those ventures in jeopardy. Health insurance industry analysts say that policy expenses for small businesses are up to 20 percent higher than those of individual consumers.

At least according to some industry experts, huge corporations face much less danger because those firms can better afford lots of policies that have high deductibles.

Also, small businesses will have a much greater per-employee administrative cost compared to huge firms. Large companies can pay for significant numbers of workers, thereby slashing the firms' overall per-employee management expenses.

These factors came to play even before the Act was approved. Employer participation varied among states. In some instances at least 95 percent of companies with more than 50 employees provided their workers with health insurance policies. That marked a sharp difference compared with small companies, only about one-third providing such coverage for employees.

Before Obamacare many smaller companies had a tougher time attracting and retaining employees than larger firms. Tiny businesses lacked the funds necessary to buy the type of good health insurance policies that lure workers to large companies.

State Exchanges Might Help Small Businesses

Those who wrote the new federal law hope that the state-run exchanges will enable employees of small companies to purchase affordable policies. Among important factors:

Job changes: People who purchase policies via the exchanges will be able to change employers without worrying whether they have complied with the mandate.

Flexibility: Many individuals buying via the exchanges will feel less "tied down" to one particular employer, which these employees otherwise would have to do just so that they could maintain coverage.

Lower incentive: Some observers worry that small employers will have less incentive to provide policies for workers because employees could buy from exchanges.

Low income: Another worry springs forth when considering the fact that small businesses will have less incentive to buy insurance for workers earning low wages.

New dilemma: Low-skilled, low-wage workers whose coverage is dropped or never offered by employers would have to get their own coverage—by joining Medicaid if they're needy and qualify, or by purchasing policies via state exchanges.

Poverty-line problems: When not covered by employers, taxpayers earning barely above poverty-line levels and who earn too much to qualify for Medicaid would be forced to buy their own policies. Deductibles could be so high that these individuals could never afford to visit a doctor, although purchasing policies as required by law.

Negative Whirlpool Effect

The Act's detrimental provisions impacting small businesses could generate a negative and irreversible "whirlpool effect" due to the countless destructive factors hidden within Obamacare.

As stated earlier, many analysts expect a large percentage of small companies to drop policies for employees at least partly as a result of the exchanges.

The tax incentives that had been designed to motivate small

companies to provide policies are only short-term, stop-gap measures. Most of these incentives are set to expire in 2015, giving such companies little or no motivation at that point to buy or continue coverage.

Some analysts view the short-term incentives as merely a diversionary tactic to prevent all small businesses from simultaneously stopping policy coverage.

The situation facing workers at small businesses will become increasingly perilous. Stress on such workers is likely to intensify if the exchanges become successful.

Small businesses would be motivated to drop coverage under such a scenario.

Beware of the Small Business Health Options Program

The crafters of Obamacare were aware of these dilemmas when writing the Act. So they also created a new bureaucracy designed to address the problem.

The Small Business Health Options Program, nicknamed "SHOP," is to start in 2017. Its goal will become to give small businesses affordable health insurance options within a specialized business healthcare exchange specifically designed for such firms.

The bureaucrats hope that SHOP will put small businesses with less than 101 employees on a level playing field with huge companies. Until now small companies have had to pay more for policies than big corporations.

SHOP's primary goals include enabling small firms to use a single exchange, thereby putting them into a single but larger risk pool. This, in turn, is designed to collectively help lower health insurance costs for small businesses.

As an added incentive, a small business that purchases policies under SHOP before the company grows to a large size could still purchase from the exchange—even after the firm eventually becomes huge.

Some analysts worry that the increased competitiveness could eventually motivate big companies to drop their policies directly, coverage that had been issued by standard insurance firms. Under worst-case scenarios this factor could eventually wreak havoc on the health insurance industry.

Deceptive Tax Incentives

Companies acquiring policies via SHOP will become eligible for potential 35-percent tax credits. Such totals would be:

Levels: Based on the amount that the firm spends to buy polices for employees.

Employee totals: This 35-percent example would be for a company with less than 11 workers.

Contribution: The firm would pay for at least 50 percent of the workers' policy premium fees.

Sliding scale: Based on a sliding scale, a lower level of credits would go to small companies employing from 11 to 25 people

Tax credit incentives such as these would vary. These benefits would be in addition to savings that officials hope that the firms will receive when buying policies via SHOP.

Under the Act's provisions at the time this book was published, in 2014 and 2015 tax credits would rise to 50 percent. Those benefits would expire in 2016, unless Congress extends such tax credits.

These convoluted and ever-changing systems had a different impact from 2010 through 2013. During that period small firms received up to 25 percent in tax credits. These totals were derived from the amounts that companies paid their workers.

Complex Regulations Spark Confusion

The confusion experienced by employees and their employers will intensify as a direct result of various quirky rules within the

Act. Among them:

Fleeing employers: Via their own free will for whatever personal reasons they choose employees can decide to buy subsidized policies from state-run exchanges, rather than join health insurance plans offered via their employers.

Employers fined: The federal government will slap fines on companies for each instance where an employee gets subsidized policies via the exchanges instead of accepting company-funded health insurance.

Retaliation prohibited: Obamacare prohibits employers from retaliating against employees for refusing company-offered policies.

Additional fines: Large companies with more than 50 employees must pay fines when the health insurance offered by the firm is deemed of "poor quality." Firms also will be fined when health insurance isn't offered to workers. Not accounting for the first 30 employees, harsh fees imposed on companies could reach $2,000 for each instance where a full-time worker uses an exchange to buy a government-subsidized policy.

The fines on companies will occur even in instances where the firms offer insurance. From the government's perspective, such instances indicate that employer-provided policies are too costly or inadequate. This confusion will intensify multi-fold, with fines set at the lesser of these totals: $3,000, for each instances were exchanges are used by employees to obtain subsidized policies; or $2,000, each instance of a full-time employee who is not given an employer-provided policy.

Senseless Monetary Fine Procedures

These goofy and arbitrary fining systems could discourage small companies from growing. Some small- or mid-size firms would risk paying $2,000 per-employee fines if the companies fail to offer health insurance, in instances where the business has at least 50 workers.

The controversy intensifies as firms argue about the definition of a "worker." Some firms are concerned that the government might arbitrarily lump seasonal or part-time employees into the definition of such a person.

Sadly, federal bureaucrats will end up making these critical decisions. The giant, self-serving and cumbersome Health and Human Services Administration will be saddled with making such determinations—perhaps involving hundreds of thousands of separate and unaffiliated companies.

Any business owner familiar with the incompetence of government cringes at this unavoidable process. Perhaps some of the biggest bloodletting will be suffered by entrepreneurs, particularly those who simultaneously own and operate numerous small businesses. The U.S. government's proverbial hammer and sickle could potentially crash down hard on such ventures in instances where the various ventures of a single entrepreneur have more than 50 employees combined.

Negatives and Positives Factors Intensify

An additional "double-edged" sword will emerge impacting small businesses and people who work at such companies.

The new provisions will make dropping health care coverage easier for small firms, which as an overall sector since 2000 have been dropping policies due to excessive costs.

This will leave the so-called "little guy" holding the bag. Employees who lose their employer-provided plans must get policies for themselves in order to comply with the mandate. The supporters of Obamacare view this as a "soft-landing process," since policies offered via the exchanges supposedly will be geared to be affordable.

Many of us who have opposed the Act from the start fear that the overall costs of policies will rise. An equal fear erupts from the burgeoning bureaucracy's built-in system of persistently slashing expenses, a pernicious process likely to steadily decrease the quality and the efficiency of health care services and products.

Critics rightfully point out that big businesses can never receive the tax credits being offered to small firms. Until now, some of the nation's largest corporations have used good health insurance policies as an enticement to prevent workers from moving to other firms. Some analysts believe lots of today's huge firms will continue to provide policies.

Yet there are many exceptions. Huge international corporations with low-paid workers such as fast-foot conglomerates do not use health insurance as a strong incentive to lure or to retain employees. Such firms have found themselves in a quandary due to recent spikes in health insurance costs, fee increases that stem directly from the various regulations imposed by Obamacare.

Brazenly showing the increasingly slimy side of American politics, the White House has issued temporary waivers at least until 2014 to various large firms within the fast-food sector. The ultimate result remains to be seen.

Eventually some huge companies may decide to completely drop all employer-provided policies, thereby agreeing to pay $2,000 per-employee fines to the government. When and if such a scenario plays out the companies likely would consider the penalties the "lesser of two evils," since finding and obtaining policies is too costly while also essentially tying up far too many corporate resources.

Russian Roulette for the American Public's Health Care

President Obama's effort to ram through at least one mindless provision of the Act got shot down by Congress in April 2011.

As originally passed by Congress and approved by the president in April 2010, the new law would have forced small businesses to file streams of useless paperwork.

Those rules would have required businesses to file 1099 forms with the IRS, keeping track of all transactions that surpassed $600. The rule also would have forced businesses to submit the same forms to people or businesses involved in those money transfers.

Socked by an onslaught of protests from businesses, a majority of congressional representatives buckled under including some Democrats who supported the original Act.

Obama felt that he had no choice other than to support the repeal of the paperwork requirement. Politicians who supported this 2011 update insisted that businesses, particularly small ventures, have better things to do than to spend a huge amount of time completing mindless and useless paperwork for the U.S. government.

Yet many average taxpayers still will suffer hardships as a direct result of the Act. Lots of people with low-pay positions, even if they work for huge corporations, are likely to lose their employer-sponsored health insurance. This will force these individuals to use their personal time and money to acquire approved policies or to join Medicaid.

All this means that Obamacare will force people to "work" during their personal time in order to satisfy Uncle Sam's socialist regulations.

Chapter 13
Summary

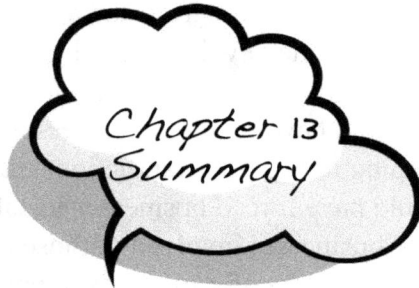

The Affordable Health Care Act will create confusion among taxpayers nationwide. Large and small businesses will have to make critical decisions on whether to provide health insurance for their employees. Many workers will unexpectedly find themselves without insurance at least temporarily. Consumers should expect lots of small companies with less than 51 employees to drop policies for their workers. All along, confusion will spring forth as many companies face fines from $2,000 to $3,000 per employee, penalties imposed for specific instances where a company fails to provide insurance for workers. Compounding these problems, streams of companies also will face fines for specific instances where the firms provide insurance but an employee chooses instead to purchase a government-subsidized policy for a state-run exchange. Meantime, streams of low-income families will start getting Medicaid coverage for the first time. Consumers should expect the overall confusion to intensify as individual states decide whether to participate in Medicaid's overall expansion.

14
State-Run Health Insurace Exchange Add to Confusion

Taxpayers nationwide should expect to undergo an extremely confusing process when forced to purchase health insurance policies from state-run exchanges.

Remember, as mentioned earlier each state will be required to operate its own health insurance exchange in time for people to complete their IRS forms in 2014. In instances where a state refuses to operate an exchange, the federal government will handle that chore.

At least judging from hundreds of news reports the vast majority of people throughout the general public seemed unaware of this process as of early 2013.

This seemed precarious since the eventual success or failure of Obamacare hinges on the efficiency of the state-run exchanges. The overall primary functions are multi-fold:

Private market: The exchanges will be designed to give people access to qualified health insurance policies offered in the private market.

Medicaid: The exchanges will give people direct links to Medicaid, in some instances letting low income people know of this system for the first time.

Inefficiencies: These systems are likely to steadily expand, to the point where employer-provided policies experience either positive or negative impacts.

Prediction: Exchanges Must be Efficient

Numerous business analysts in recent years have insisted that Obamacare will evolve into a dismal failure if the exchanges are inefficient.

The exchanges will not be as simple as some supporters of the Act want consumers to believe. Using devious propaganda techniques, these bureaucrats and politicians equate the exchanges to giant department stories where consumers go to shop.

Under this line of thinking, when shopping for policies consumers will be able to pick and choose their favorites in much the same way that they compare home products.

Yet a grim reality forces many of us who believe that some consumers will have a difficult time making these critical choices. Certainly, buying a health insurance policy is far more confusing and intricate than choosing which coffee maker to buy. As a result consumers will need to face a variety of critical and sometimes complex choices:

Subsidies: When you enter a department store, government workers do not hand you piles of cash to assist you in making your purchases. Yet that's essentially a possibility for low-income consumers when they're reviewing options at a state-run exchange.

Qualify: Many people likely will have difficulty determining whether they qualify for government subsidies. Getting government assistance on a sliding scale will hinge on how much income the person earns during a calendar year.

Incomes vary: Some people have sharply fluctuating incomes, earning far more in some years than in others. Thus, some people might qualify for subsidies one year, while getting no government assistance the next. This will make budget planning difficult.

Defiance: Angered by the challenging regulations imposed by Obamacare, some states have indicated their potential refusal to start and run exchanges. As previously mentioned, the federal bureaucracy will start and operate exchanges for states refusing to participate.

Rebellion: As reported by the "Washington Post," as of February 2013 the U.S. government planned to operate the exchanges of more than half of the 50 states—at least 26 of them by the latest count. The deadline for states to declare whether they would comply was Feb. 15, 2013. In addition to the 26 states that refused to join, seven states decided to partner with the U.S. government in sharing responsibility for their exchanges.

Most States Rejected Obamacare Exchanges

The startling development of the defiance of most states received little if any coverage in the mainstream liberal news media. Yet this "silent rebellion" could emerge as a considerable setback to the government's bureaucratic plans.

A handful of states that favor Democrats refused to participate, and a small number of Republican-leaning states decided to operate exchanges. A "Washington Post" analysis showed that the split either for or against the state-by-state exchange system generally followed party lines.

Thus, the U.S. map depicting states that refused and those that joined generally mirrors the Electoral College results shown on presidential election nights. For the most part a huge swath of middle-America has refused to participate in the exchanges.

Clearly, a majority of Americans still oppose Obamacare, which these individuals feel as if they're being forced to buy something against their will. Even some high-population states including Florida and Ohio that voted for Obama in November 2012 refused to launch state-run exchanges.

Combined and individually, these factors clearly show that the United States as a whole is perhaps more politically divided than ever. Whether this bodes well for the long-term success of Obamacare has yet to be seen.

If the past is used as any indication, once Americans receive a federal entitlement such as Social Security they become politically ferocious—especially whenever anyone threatens to take away such benefits. Over time, if Obamacare continues to limp along at even a mediocre success increasing numbers of people are likely to vehemently support the program politically, even if they're unaware of the damage the ill-advised law inflicts upon the medical industry and upon the economy.

Learn of the Act's Many Flaws

Contrary to what many supporters of Obamacare might tell the public, the Act features numerous "soft spots" that could generate significant problems for the public.

Essentially thumbing their noses at consumers nationwide, political cronies insist that both Democrats and Republicans like the exchanges—although such assessments often fall far from reality. Among key challenges:

Consumer issues: The political lobbyists and politicians who crafted the legislation insist that the new rules protect consumers. These analysts claim that in order to be certified by the government, the plans must provide what bureaucrats label as essential guarantees regarding public health. However, these loosely defined regulations fail to ensure that the best, cutting-edge services will be available. To the contrary, via IPAB and other processes based on cronyism, the system will continually strive to slash what the government is willing to pay for specific services— thereby minimizing quality.

More choices: Many of them fully believing their own propaganda, the Act's supporters claim that the exchanges will give consumers more choices among numerous qualified health insurance plans. However, some observers note that states with low populations will have less competition among health insurance companies. This, in turn, could result in sharply higher policy premium prices within those states. Meantime, consumers in highly populous regions might have to choose from a lengthy maze of confusing or highly complex plans. Some insurance companies might be far stronger or much more reliable than others. Yet from viewing the exchanges consumers would have little or no way of accessing such critical details.

Equality: Obamacare supporters claim that the system will require that all insurance companies provide equal levels of coverage on a tiered basis. While such efforts might seem commendable at first glance, once again the quality and reliability of individual insurance companies will not be listed within the exchanges. Companies with poor records of paying for patients' costs or that require excessive unnecessary paperwork would not be listed within the exchanges as having "bad marks." Could this be because insurance industry lobbyists played a significant role in writing the legislation?

Lack of competition: Supporters of the Act like to say that the exchanges will significantly ramp up competition among insurance companies. This supposedly would occur because in some cases millions of consumers would be reviewing the state exchanges in hopes of getting the best "deals." Of course, only "time will tell," since Obamacare would have to remain in full force until the results of such assumptions are known. Even before Obamacare went into full force, during 2011 and 2012, and well into 2013, consumers who had been purchasing their own policies began to complain that the insurance firms were indiscriminately raising rates. If the more-competition theory were correct, why did prices price increase? Just as distressing, what would prevent additional cost jumps after the exchanges launch?

Government Incompetence Will Accelerate

The exchanges will shoot the state and federal bureaucracies into overdrive. When using this process, consumers will be able to review options and purchase policies in a variety of ways:

Online: Via the official, government-authorized Website of the state where the consumer lives.

Personal service: Directly in person at "brick-and-mortar" offices inside the state where the person lives. Some observers equate such facilities to the Department of Motor Vehicles or DMV offices already operated by state governments.

Phone service: Consumers will be able to access or acquire policies via toll-free telephone numbers, verbally ordering policies over the phone.

With so many options, many people might think that the new system will quickly emerge as easy for consumers to access and to understand. To the contrary, however, many low-income consumers lack Internet access or don't even own phones.

Just as distressing, think of what it's like to visit a DMV office. The mere thought of such a process leaves a sour taste in the mouths of many people being forced into Obamacare. Even the "New York Times," which has an undisputed history as a champion of liberal causes, said in late 2012 that operating an exchange is an "immense technical challenge requiring sophistical information technology." Such an integral system would be needed, the newspaper said, to digest and display huge amounts of data, listing the costs and benefits of each insurance plan.

Hoping to skirt such issues, some observers have even posed the question of whether the public would be better served by a single national exchange operated by the federal government. Yet from the perspective of many Internet technology experts the U.S. government has been a dismal failure in forming and operating Web-based systems. Streams of news reports through the first 13 years of the 21st Century chronicled numerous incidents where U.S. government Websites were hacked or compromised.

Most People Currently Dislike These Senseless Provisions

Understandably, national public opinion polls consistently indicate that many Americans perceive Obamacare as essentially "big-brother run amuck."

At least from the view of many citizens, the out-of-control federal bureaucracy has no right to make such critical decisions regarding their lives. And, now that there is no way for the average citizen to stop Obamacare due to the Supreme Court's ruling, many citizens seem doubly wary about the notion of a single, unified national health exchange.

Adding to the confusion, each state has its own regulations regarding health insurance. These individualized rules that vary from state-to-state regulate everything from consumer rights to what is expected of insurance companies. For instance, state-imposed insurance rules in Alabama are likely far different from those in California.

Largely for these reasons, some people might understandably become wary of any one-size-fits-all strategy in potentially developing a single unified national exchange.

Any citizen who has ever had to deal with problems related to the IRS knows that getting a final answer or resolution to a dispute can sometimes take many years. What should be done to convince consumers that state-run exchanges or even a single national exchange would be any more efficient?

In order to bolster or to legitimize their efforts, some proponents of Obamacare have noted that much if its regulations were molded after Massachusetts' state-mandated health care system.

Developed under the administration of former Governor Mitt Romney, a Republican, the Bay State legislation requires citizens to have health insurance policies. Some politicians deemed the Massachusetts Health Connector program as so successful that some states have modeled their exchanges after that system. Yet adversaries of that program claim it has significantly lowered disposable incomes of households in that state, while pumping up health insurance costs and resulting in job losses.

Chapter 14 Summary

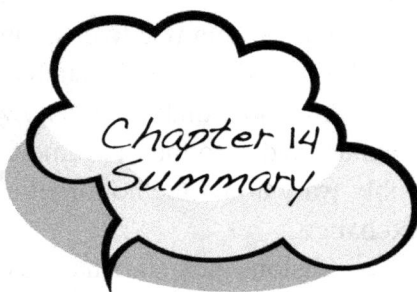

Already a dismal failure from its inception, the Affordable Health Care Act is expected to leave more than 19 million Americans without health insurance in 2019, according to estimates by the non-partisan Congressional Budget Office. More than half of the 50 states have refused to participate in the state-run exchanges due largely to obvious flaws within Obamacare. Many people will have difficulty accessing state-run exchanges. There is no guarantee that insurance companies listed via those services in physical offices, on Websites and via toll-free numbers will promptly pay legitimate insurance claims. Only insurance companies that have been approved by the cumbersome federal bureaucracy will be included in each state's exchange. Obamacare supporters insist that this process will minimize insurance bills. Yet many monthly insurance premiums purchased individually by consumers already sustained steep annual increases in 2012 and 2013, even before Obamacare was to click into full gear.

15

The Fallacy of "Essential Health Benefits"

As initially enacted Obamacare requires that an insurance company must provide "essential health benefits" before such policies can be listed as qualified.

Par for the course, however, well into 2013 the bureaucrats in Washington, D.C., still had not clearly defined what this is supposed to mean. Thus, just before the Affordable Health Care Act was "set to sail," the new rules had already become a rudderless ship.

Rushed to meet the 2014 deadline, the cumbersome and sometimes inept U.S. Department of Health and Human Services still needed to bandage a hodgepodge of regulations together. The agency was assigned the formidable task of determining the specific criteria that the insurance companies must meet in order to become certified.

If the past is any indication of future strategies, lobbyists for the insurance agencies likely would assist the agency in defining "essential health benefits." Predictably the insurance industry essentially would be crafting the rules of regulations to meet its own needs, rather than looking out for the best interests of consumers.

As mentioned earlier, the exchanges will list policies within four standardized plan categories—platinum, gold, silver and bronze. The so-called higher platinum levels do not necessarily relate to a better quality of health care, but rather lower deductibles.

All levels from bronze to platinum will offer at least some plans that require out-of-pocket expenses or deductibles that consumers must pay each year toward their own health care. For instance, a person with a subsidized policy needing $127,000 in medical care during one calendar year would have to pay a maximum deductible.

The specific amount that the person must pay will depend on the percentage of costs paid for by the type of plan the patient acquired. The percentage of deductible costs covered by each plan would differ on a sliding scale. Percentages mentioned as possibilities have included; bronze, 60 percent of deductibles; silver, 70 percent; gold, 80 percent; and platinum, 90 percent.

Will Bureaucrats Protect Consumers?

The deductible structures on sliding scales are only one part of a maze of options likely to confuse average citizens. Consumers nationwide must face a lengthy list of other features packed onto the legislation by bureaucrats. Among these features:

Income: Whenever people want to apply for government-funded subsidies to help pay for their policies acquired via exchanges, they'll need to carefully review an endless labyrinth of sliding fee scales. All options will hinge on the person's income. Then, the total amount of subsidies that a person qualifies for will hinge on how his or her income—or their combined family's income—ranks within the "federal poverty level."

Federal Poverty Level: The official United States "poverty level" is set annually by bureaucrats who work for the U.S. Department of Health and Human Services.

Qualification: The percentage that the U.S. government will pay for a family will be hooked to a sliding scale. The highest percentages of subsidy payments will go to the poorest families, while those earning more will have to pay higher percentages of premium costs. A four-person family earning less than 400 percent of the poverty level can qualify for at least some government subsidies when purchasing via the exchanges.

Out-of-pocket expenses: Also based on the individual's income level coupled with the federal poverty level, each consumer shopping at the exchange can review potential options that might lower out-of-pocket expenses. These are fees or "deductibles" that policy holders must pay before an insurance company starts covering medical costs.

Premium levels: These are the amounts that a policy holder must pay to an insurance company every month in order to maintain coverage. Once again, the government will subsidize a percentage of these fees to qualified taxpayers based on their incomes as compared to where their family falls within the poverty level.

Basic Health Plans: Adding to the confusion, Obamacare gives every state an option to create what the federal paper-pushers call a "basic health plan." These would be set up for individuals with low incomes. As usual the federal regulations here are pegged at percentage levels of the federal poverty line that some people might consider arbitrary. As of 2010 these would have been for individuals earning $14,400 to $21,660, their incomes from 133 percent to 200 percent of that year's poverty level. The bureaucrats require that basic health plans feature all essential benefits offered in qualified platinum, gold, silver and bronze policies.

Actuarial value: Those who embrace the Act's many convoluted requirements insist that the new system's goals of lowering out-of-pocket expenses and decreasing premiums will pump up the "actuarial value" of what the government spends. For each specific policy, this term is used by bureaucrats as a way of insisting that the government will pay a higher share of medical expenses for poor people than for those earning more. Once again, this is merely political double-speak, covering up the fact that Americans who strive to succeed financially will be forced to buy all or at least some of the medical insurance given to the poor.

Cumbersome Government "Quality" Standards

Eager to sidestep potential criticism that this hodgepodge of rules lacks any "checks and balances" that would assure good-quality insurance, the bureaucrats set up a list of standards that such companies must meet. Once again, here we have an instance of lobbyists helping to craft legislation that would regulate an industry that they represent.

This façade that attempts to mimic reliable regulation hinges on "performance metrics" that the political cronies and politicians have authorized. In terms that average people might better understand this means that the bureaucrats decided to rate the performance or quality of an insurance company and an insurance policy on:

Denials: The number of a policy-holder claims that that the insurance company denies.

Drop outs: The total of people who leave a specific policy offered by the insurance company.

Excessive numbers in either or both of these primary categories supposedly signifies a company or a policy that fails to meet standards that insurance sellers should meet.

Yet those of us wary about the effectiveness of Obamacare view these supposed standards as mere window dressing. In a sense this is like viewing an old vintage car. The vehicle might look spiffy and shiny from the outside, while the engine fails to run with any degree of efficiency.

Ultimately the question that consumers to ask themselves in this regard is: "Why would insurance companies help develop regulations that ultimately would cause themselves damage and a loss of potential revenue?"

With this at the front of our minds, many of us with the good sense to remain wary of the Act expect a handful of these companies to get dinged on occasion as a mere "window-dressing" procedure. We fear such instances would occur only in a phony effort to pretend society has an efficient regulatory system.

Many of us are concerned that the insurance industry and the government will view the general public as "gullible" regarding the standards. The levels of "drop-outs" and "denied claims" supposedly serves as a spyglass affording a clear view into whether insurance companies: make purchasing policies easy; help policy holders get answers or resolutions to their concerns; and also how well the companies give consumers access to "adequate" health care services.

Some Lawmakers Launched a Diversionary Tactic

Apparently aware of Obamacare's countless flaws, in January 2013 numerous Democrats in the House of Representatives within Congress proposed what they labeled as the "Public Option Deficit Reduction Act." With Congresswoman Janice Schakowsky, an Illinois Democrat as a main sponsor, the bill was introduced in conjunction with 43 other House members. According to various news reports, the non-partisan government agencies that analyze and forecast federal finances:

Obamacare: Would add $6.2 trillion to the U.S. government's long-term deficit, according to a General Accounting Office analysis released in February 2013 in the "National Review" and other news publications.

Public option: Under representative Schakowsky's proposal to make national health care a public option, the U.S. government's public debt would decrease $104 billion over a 10-year period, according to Congressional Budget Office estimates reported in "The Hill" publication in January 2013.

As proposed by Schakowsky and the bill's other sponsors the Public Option Deficit Reduction Act would amend Obamacare by creating a "public option."

According to the Schakowsky bill's official summary published by the federal government's Library of Congress, the Secretary of Health and Human Services would be required to offer "through the exchanges a health benefit plan (public health insurance option) that ensures choice, competition and stability of affordable, high-quality coverage throughout the United States." The library's official summary also states that the secretary's primary responsibility would be to create a low-cost plan without compromising quality and access to care.

At face value, all this might sound admirable. But the legislation likely needs much more thorough analysis in order to determine whether this proposed revision to the Act approved in 2010 would ultimately hurt or help health care and the health insurance industry within the United States.

Is This a Strategy to Completely Socialize Health Care?

The term "public option" within the title of Schakowsky's bill likely will ignite fears that her proposed revisions would result in a system as inept as that used in Canada.

Dubbed as a "public option" system that relies on a "single-payer" process, the Canadian system does not charge that nation's citizens directly for health care.

While such a system might seem admirable, by many accounts the Canadian program is a dismal failure. Patients across that nation often have to wait many months or even years to receive basic health treatments or services, reportedly even in certain life-threatening situations.

The problem north of the U.S. borders has gotten so bad, according to many news reports, that streams of Canadians often flock to the United States for basic health procedures and treatments.

A cursory review of Schakowsky's plan fails to indicate whether that proposal would essentially put the U.S. government in full charge of health care for all citizens. That is not the case under Obamacare, at least from the view of many of its advocates. From their view under the current Act the country's insurance companies and health treatment providers still compete—thereby theoretically resulting in lower overall prices.

According to the Library of Congress report, the Illinois congresswoman's proposal would require that the new public health insurance option:

Availability: Only be made available to the public via the exchanges.

Regulations: Must comply with requirements applicable to other health benefit plans offered through such exchanges. These features would include requirements relates to benefits, benefit levels, provider networks, notices, consumer protections and cost sharing.

Features: Must offer bronze, silver and gold plan levels.

A potential danger looms that these features would contribute even more to the ever-growing bureaucratic maze regarding health care within the United States. The increasingly complex and difficult-to-map cobweb of rules might become even more difficult to manage, while contributing to public misunderstandings about what is offered.

Making Americans Dependant Upon Government

Although Schakowsky's intentions might be admirable, with little doubt her proposal would make Americans increasingly dependent on health care decisions made by government bureaucrats. Her legislation also proposes that:

Ombudsman: The Secretary of Health and Human Services would bulk up that already oversized federal agency to include an ombudsman to oversee the "public health insurance option."

Information: "Collect such data as may be required to establish premiums and payment rates."

Regions: Establish "geographically adjusted premiums at a level fully sufficient to finance the costs of the health benefits provided and administrative costs related to the operation of the plan."

Charges: Establish payment rates and provide for greater payment rates for the first three years.

At first glance these various proposals seem to be a rehash of controversial "public option" efforts proposed by Democrats in 2010 around the time Obamacare won congressional approval. Opponents of that provision had argued that a government-run health insurance plan would have stifled competition among insurance providers.

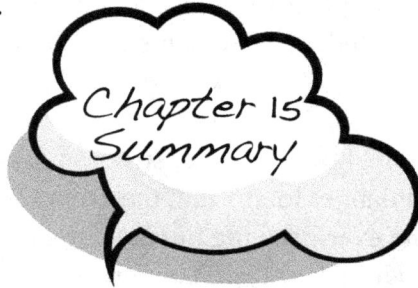

Chapter 15 Summary

As approved by Congress in 2010, the Affordable Health Care Act required that health insurance companies maintain "essential health benefits." Yet three years later in 2013 as Obamacare was poised to click into the first phase of full gear, the federal bureaucrats still had not compiled those definitions. A danger loomed that insurance company lobbyists would work behind the scenes to craft the eventual rules to their employers' own benefit. Meantime, the expected fees that consumers would have to pay and federal subsidies on a sliding scale generated a hodgepodge of difficult-to-understand fee levels. The legislation as proposed fails to safeguard the public interest, other than launching a lame system that rates insurance company policies within the exchanges based on how many claims are denied and also on the number of people dropping specific policies. Potentially compounding these problems and adding even more confusion to an already perplexing situation, an Illinois congresswoman has proposed an amendment to Obamacare that could eventually open a gateway to a full-scale takeover by the U.S. government of the insurance and health care industries—potentially eliminating competition within those business sectors, ultimately raising prices.

16

Expect Rapidly Increasing Costs

Obamacare means "bad news" for anyone striving to save money, especially those among the hard-working and ever-shrinking American middle-class.

A wide variety of economists and health industry analysts expect overall health care costs to continue to skyrocket upward in the foreseeable future. Consumers should expect such increases on the heels of already harsh jumps in such fees during the first decade of the 21st Century.

Those who support Obamacare like to breeze past the cost issue. Instead, they often like to focus all their attention on the apparent fact that many Americans for the first time will begin receiving health insurance coverage.

Lots of observers seem to agree that the Act will achieve its admirable goal of giving more people access to health insurance coverage. The expansion of Medicaid and the state-by-state exchanges featuring government subsidies for those who qualify should play a significant role.

Yet in all likelihood overall health care costs should continue to jump. Among primary reasons:

Life expectancies: Americans are living far longer than average citizens did during the early 19th Century or even just 50 years ago.

Surging elderly: Along with increases in the time people are expected to live, the senior population will surge to all-time highs as the Baby Boom generation passes middle-age.

Critical resources: One of the overall population's fastest-growing segments, these elderly will put a burden on already limited health care resources nationwide.

Pivotal time: This growth in the elderly population will come during the critical period where the U.S. government strives to cut back on health care services and related expenses involving seniors—all done, ironically, in an effort to minimize costs.

Technology: Health care industry analysts insist that the technology used in the U.S. market is far more advanced than in most other countries. But the so-called tradeoff comes at a significant price, as Americans pay much more than people in most other countries for health insurance and also for specific treatments rarely made available elsewhere.

Life Expectancy Plays a Critical Role

Many people rightfully criticize the U.S. health care system. They point out that although the overall American life expectancy has increased markedly, according to United Nations data the United States ranked 40th worldwide in that category in 2010.

The many other so-called lesser-developed nations ranking above the USA in the life-expectancy rankings included numerous nations with nationalized health insurance—including: Taiwan, 39th; Denmark, 38th, Cuba, 37th; the United Kingdom, 23rd; and even Canada, 11th.

The vast majority of national-run or government-operated systems in countries other than the United States are dismal failures, at least according to a wide variety of news reports. Even so, at least one of them, the nationalized, tax-subsidized health care system in Denmark is efficient, at least according to Christopher Rosenmeier, a post-doctoral fellow at the University of Cambridge and a scholar of modern Chinese literature.

Writing a column for the "Denver Post," Rosenmeier, a native of Denmark, cited an international survey that concluded at least 90 percent of Danes "are totally satisfied with their health care, and it uses the most advanced methods available anywhere. And per-capita, there are more doctors and hospital beds than in the U.S.

"It's mainly cheap because it's a lot simpler to manage. There are no medical insurance companies or lawyers operating for profit, or financial background checks. There are no uninsured, so there is no paperwork if you get sick or injured."

Even if Rosenmeier's assumptions are correct, that doesn't take away the fact that the overall American system is bloated with inflated costs—unable to match the prices and quality of healthcare in his homeland.

Meantime, streams of people living in countries other than the United States might enjoy far greater life expectancies thanks largely to the fact that they enjoy healthier lifestyles and eat better foods than Americans.

U.S. Healthcare Expenses Skyrocket

In 2008, the last full calendar year for which statistics were available in 2013, the United States spent a whopping 15.2 percent of the nation's gross domestic profit on healthcare. That's $7,146 per capita, and those totals are now likely closer to 17 percent of U.S. GDP, according to the World Health Organization and other groups.

Sadly, however, according to a National Institutes of Health report in 2013, among 17 high-income countries studied the United States ranked near last in numerous vital medical categories. These included heart and lung disease, homicides, infant mortality, adolescent pregnancies, and injuries.

The magnitude of the problems facing the U.S. healthcare industry is worsened by the greed of Big Pharma, a nickname for the pharmaceutical industry. Empowered by high-paid political lobbyists and seedy connections with Congress, Big Pharma gouges the American public by dramatically increasing the prices of drugs sold domestically. The devastation becomes even more evident as the same companies often sell identical pharmaceutical products much cheaper in other countries that have nationalized healthcare.

The Affordable Health Care Act drastically worsens this situation on everything from drugs to basic medical products and treatments that consumers need. Rather than concentrating the bulk of its efforts to keep drug costs at reasonable levels, Obamacare's primary efforts focus on expanding the bureaucracy in an effort to serve more people.

Bowing to pressure from consumers, the new rules force insurance companies to accept patients who suffer from pre-existing medical conditions. These regulations also prohibit the corporations from charging such individuals more than healthy people for policies. As a result, the insurance companies will have to pay significantly more in medical fees than if such individuals had been banned from the process.

As previously mentioned, to enable insurance companies to remain viable, those who wrote the legislation essentially covered up this flaw by forcing healthy people—many who previously lacked health care insurance—to buy or to obtain such policies.

Destructive Measures Grew

Overly eager to essentially "give away the farm," the creators of Obamacare added more destructive measures that resulted in increased costs. Some critics called these additional provisions "runaway socialism," while the Act's supporters called these regulations essential in order to provide adequate health care services for all Americans. Among some of the worst, most destructive cost-increasing requirements:

Caps: Eliminated financial limits on the amounts that insurance companies would have to pay for an individual's health care services during a single year.

Lifetime: Enacted a potentially reckless rule that forced the insurance firms to remove the "caps" or total lifetime expenditures on any single individual.

Young adults: As previously mentioned, for the first time all general policies allowed parents to retain coverage for their children up to age 26.

Blanket coverage: Also as stated earlier, the insurance companies would for the first time have to cover all "essential health benefits"—which the government needs to define.

Losses: The new rule tightens "medical loss ratios," a term that essentially means insurance companies now have less wiggle room to earn as much profit as possible. For instance, an insurance company that pays out $67 in claims for every $100 that it collects has a 67 percent loss ratio. The Act "tightens" these margins, limiting potential profits. Critics allege that this "loss ratio" restriction puts pressure on insurance companies to raise policy prices, in order to offset any high payments to doctors and healthcare firms.

Sticking It to the Little Guy

Remember, insurance company lobbyists and their crony politicians actually helped craft these restrictions. So, why did the firms agree to these potentially cost-increasing measures?

They were collectively able to "stick it to the little guy," forcing the average consumer to purchase health insurance policies even among consumers who don't want them. Partly to make this happen, the devilish insiders who crafted the legislation also took great care to avoid including any restrictions on cost increases.

This back-room skullduggery enabled them to set in place a mandatory process that would pump an additional 30 million more customers onto the insurance company rolls.

From the perspective of insurance companies, an added

financial benefit comes in the form of the government-paid subsidies—where Uncle Sam helps cover the insurance premium bills of qualified low-income people who purchase policies via the exchanges.

Essentially, the lobbyists and Obamacare supporters crafted a corrupt, self-serving back-room deal that was self-serving for their own political and financial needs. The big losers, of course, were the American public in general—but who really cared about those people?

Understandably angry that the Act was being forced upon them, many frustrated Americans sat by helplessly as continual news reports chronicled how people would be forced to buy insurance. On the other side of the political aisle many consumers were cheering, including individuals with pre-existing medical conditions and lots of those with low incomes.

It wasn't until nearly three years after the corrupt Congress passed the Act that many consumers for the first time began to realize the "error of their ways." Lots of people who had previously supported the measure without knowing what the legislation entailed finally began protesting—claiming the rules were too expensive or not good enough.

Slimy Politics Prevailed

Slimy politics greased up the works within three years after Congress passed the Act in April 2010. The Obama administration issued more than 2,000 waivers to its political cronies through November 2012. This corrupt process allowed hand-picked companies and labor unions to avoid the new health care law's harsh provisions.

According to a report by Michelle Malkin at "National Review Online," among the first and most prominent recipients of the Obamacare waivers "were large restaurant chains that provide low-wage, seasonal and part-time workers" with low-cost insurance policies called "mini-med" plans.

As explained by Malkin, an estimated "1.7 million workers benefit from such plans. Obamacare forced companies carrying such coverage to raise their coverage limits to no less than $750,000 annually. Another Obamacare provision forces all insurers to spend at least 80 percent to 85 percent of their premiums on medical care."

The long, grimy hands of people crafting the rules used the legislation in an effort to dictate more than merely health care. Rather than just managing insurance coverage amounts, their goal was to dictate "marketing, salaries and other costs," Malkin said. "The regulation punished (the) companies mini-med plans whose insurers' high administrative costs were due to frequent worker turnover and relatively low spending on claims—not 'greed.'" Malkin was among analysts who concluded that tens of thousands of workers would lose their healthcare insurance due to the regulations.

Many of these waivers allowing firms to avoid Obamacare rules were granted by the fall of 2010. Yet by late 2012 and early 2013 lots of major fast food chains including McDonald's and Darden Restaurants—which operates many franchises including Red Lobster and Oliver Garden—considered moving full-time workers to less than 30 hours per week. That way, the companies hoped, they could avoid falling under Obamacare's provisions at the time when additional phases of the Act started being implemented.

Thus, perhaps hundreds of thousands of hardworking Americans will have their incomes negatively impacted. An undeniable fact began to emerge. Rather than merely striving to help people in need of health care, Obamacare was actually beginning to wreak havoc on the American economy. The "do-gooder" and "help-everyone" mindset threatened to undermine the very fabric of American business and entrepreneurialism.

Many Hard-Working Consumers Will Suffer While "Lazy People" Benefit

As a prime example, consider the plight of a theoretical family in the United States. Here are the health care stories of two people in that close-knit group.

Dwight: He earns $35,000 yearly mowing lawns at age 56. Since his income is barely within pre-designated multiples of the official U.S. poverty level, Dwight must purchase his own health insurance policy in order to satisfy the new Obamacare mandate. As a result, he spends $200 monthly to purchase a required policy. Yet barely earning enough money to live, Dwight is unable to visit the doctor whenever seriously ill because he cannot afford to pay for medical costs other than co-pays. The situation got so bad that Dwight was unable to visit a doctor after developing what physicians call "adult on-set stuttering," an extremely rare medical condition. Physicians say such rare stuttering that suddenly starts during adulthood is often considered an early warning sign of a brain tumor, a recent stroke or early symptoms of Parkinson's disease. Like most Americans in today's sluggish economy Dwight needed to continue working although his medical condition worsened. He earned too much to apply for Medicaid or to qualify for government subsidies to his health insurance payments. "Being forced to buy health insurance is tantamount to me being required to literally throw my hard-earned money out of a window, in the form of mandatory insurance premiums that I can never use," Wayne said. "I get nothing in return for my expenses."

Barbara: Dwight's 41-year-old step-daughter recently got laid off from her job as a manager at a high-end wine store. Unmarried, Barbara started living with her boyfriend, a successful businessman in his mid-30s. Deeply in love with the man and being cared for by him, Barbara decided to return to school attending only two classes a week—a writing class just for fun. Feeling no need to find work, she applied for and was accepted into Medicaid as one of its fully-qualified participants. As a result, Barbara was able to get all of her medical needs paid for, and she never needs to fork out a single cent for monthly premiums, for co-payments or for deductibles.

Jose: At age 37 he snuck illegally into the United States from Mexico in 2010. Then, in 2013 he suffered a heart attack that left him disabled. Beginning in 2014, hard-working American citizens who earn middle-class or high-end incomes will have to start paying for Jose's medical care although he has never paid a penny to the U.S. government.

Frank: At age 26 in 2009, Frank robbed a bank in Fort Myers, Florida, shortly before being shot by police who were protecting themselves after he fired upon them. An officer's bullet shattered Frank's spine, leaving him disabled. After Frank is released from prison in 2015, he will be able to qualify as a Medicaid recipient, and thereafter hard-working and law-abiding Americans will have to pay this man's medical expenses for the remainder of his life.

Under Obamacare, many hard-working individuals will be forced to buy policies without getting any substantive health care. Others who choose to avoid working or who have broken the law will get streams of health care benefits, which will continue as long as they remain unemployed or manage to earn just enough to remain qualify for Medicaid.

Of course, there are exceptions, positive stories of truly needy people who are getting coverage for the first time. Other success stories involve people who can finally receive coverage because health insurance companies no longer can refuse policies to individuals with pre-existing medical conditions.

The liberal mainstream media chooses to tell the admirable stories of these needy people finally getting medical help. Yet sadly the plights of the countless people whose predicaments are similar to Dwight's are being fully ignored in the mainstream news.

Criminals, Illegal Aliens and Drug Addicts Will Benefit

People who should be delighted by Obamacare's provisions include drug addicts, those who drive recklessly and even bank robbers who get shot while in the act of administering their crimes. While millions of individuals like Dwight are required by the new law to pay for their insurance but cannot afford to see a doctor, streams of narcotics abusers and low-income drunken drivers injured in wrecks due to their own careless behavior will have to pay little if anything.

From the view of many observers, everything comes down to a question of political ideology. Among key factors to consider are "what is fair? And, is it okay to force healthy, hard-working and industrious people to essentially pay for the health care of people who choose not to work, who lack ambition and those who want the government to essentially do everything for them?

"Perhaps just as important, is it fair and all right to force people to buy something that they don't want or that they don't feel they can afford?"

Well, to many people the answers to all these questions might be "yes," while other individuals might give a resounding "no." Still other observers would give varying answers, or they might lack any opinion.

Yet at least one thing is for sure. Whether we like the Obamacare system or not, the answers have essentially all been made for us by politicians. Clearly stated, the time for asking such questions has passed us by because Congress has enacted this ill-advised legislation.

Moving forward, the key issues will focus on whether the Act can be modified, and also what specific changes if any should be made. Many political analysts say that the possibility of repealing Obamacare is almost non-existent, particularly during the president's second four-year term, which ends in January 2017.

Political Minefield

The various complex provisions of Obamacare have created a political minefield. The proverbial landscape just up ahead for the American public is hidden with buried "financial bombs." Remember, as stated earlier, the non-partisan U.S. General Accounting Office has projected that Obamacare will add $6.2 trillion in long-term debt to the federal government.

As the current decade ends and the 2020s click into gear, the financial impacts of Obamacare on federal, state and local governments will become increasingly clear.

By then, unless Obamacare is drastically revised in the interim, the fiscal train will be chugging ahead full speed at too fast a pace to even try to stop.

Hopefully, the potential financial Armageddon sparked by the Act and the nation's other economic problems will stop short of generating a second Great Depression.

Numerous economists warn that such an outcome is inevitable, while others insist that such worries are pure nonsense. Whatever the case, at least judging by what numerous financial experts have proclaimed so far the nation's economic woes will become even more challenging.

On the positive side, at least in the short-term, the Act has done wonders for at least some families. Starting in the early fall of 2010, health insurance companies no longer were able to deny coverage to children who suffered from pre-existing medical problems. Sadly, however, apparently due to the vast quagmire of loopholes in Obamacare, some health insurance companies managed to sidestep those regulations. Rather than face such expenses until fully required to beginning in January 2014, some insurance companies simply stopped selling insurance plans that covered just children but not their families.

Chapter 16
Summary

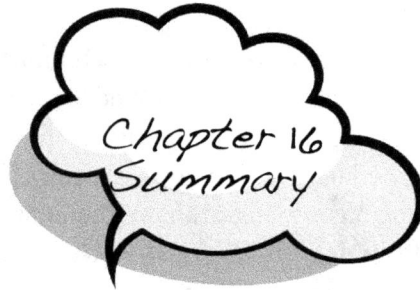

Overall health care costs and health insurance policy premiums are likely to continue increasing nationwide despite Obamacare. In fact, many of these jumps in fees are likely to occur as a direct and indirect result of the Act. The new rules have numerous stipulations that analysts universally believe will push up costs to consumers, to insurance companies and to health care providers. Among key factors in pushing up costs are provisions requiring insurance companies to give unlimited lifetime benefits on health care coverage and a rule that those firms also remove any caps on their annual expenses. The public remains angry at these price increases but average citizens can do nothing to significantly lower the overall costs of health care providers, the government and insurance companies. On the positive side, the new rules will enable millions of people to get health insurance coverage for the first time. Even so, lots of hard-working individuals will be forced to buy policies that they can never use, unable to afford deductibles. Despite the Act's many pitfalls lots of people appreciate the new rules and they also accept this political ideology. Streams of other Americans take a completely opposite opinion. Economists project that the Affordable Health Care Act will increase the federal government's debt by $6.2 trillion.

17
Growing Bureaucracy Equals Increased Inefficiencies

In the eyes of many observers, Obamacare is worse than an unstoppable, fast-approaching level-five hurricane with the most powerful potential destruction imaginable.

The fundamental element of Obamacare robs power from "doctors, patients, and even insurance companies, and transfers the power to the federal government," political analyst Dick Morris wrote in an online commentary in February 2013.

Morris tells Americans to avoid believing the "Obama propaganda that the new law won't change anything in your personal health care universe. It will in reality change everything."

Among some of the changes mentioned most frequently by critics of the Act:

Fewer Doctors: The nation will have tens of thousands fewer doctors than needed, according to the Association of American Medical Colleges. Critics argue that many potential medical students will avoid the profession rather than face bureaucratic issues.

Fleeing Industry: An estimated 360,000 physicians may leave the medical industry, unwilling to adapt to the changes, according to reports issued by "Investors Business Daily." Along with the decrease in medical students, this would worsen the doctor shortage.

Age squeeze: People between ages 55 and 65 might face

potential problems if they retire early. Obamacare supposedly has stop-gap measures designed to entice employers to cover these individuals until their Medicare eligibility kicks in at age 65. The bureaucrats call this a "reinsurance" program. But some observers worry that in the scramble for affordable coverage, such individuals might get overlooked.

Hating physicians: Piling on the damage from the view of some doctors, the new rules also hamper the efforts of physician-owned medical facilities or hospitals. Starting in 2010, the Act stopped such facilities from participating in Medicare—considered an essential revenue source for any hospital to remain viable. Although some exemptions to this mindless rule remain possible, consumers should expect the growth of physician-owned hospitals to fade or stop.

War on Private Enterprise: The rules also discourage or hamper a competitive free-market system that might tend to drive down prices. Rather than relying on private business, the big-spending politicians—overly eager to fork out tax dollars and bloat the bureaucracy—devised a way to fund "community health centers nationwide." Under provisions of the Act, the federal government will subsidize these facilities in rural communities or inner-cities neighborhoods where bureaucrats conclude that far too many people remain without health insurance despite Obamacare. The federal government must spend an estimated $11 billion to build this infrastructure, designed in part to serve illegal immigrants who have unlawfully snuck into the United States—individuals who would not otherwise qualify for such government-funded healthcare.

Obamacare Wages War Against Physicians

Whether the politicians and lobbyists who devised Obamacare admit this, their scheme has collectively "declared war" on physicians in the United States.

Sadly, this development comes at a pivotal time in scientific research where doctors have been on the verge of devising significant potential advancements in patient care.

Rather than focusing the bulk of their efforts on such significant and essential goals, many doctors now will have to spend increasing amounts of time and resources complying with the burgeoning federal bureaucracy.

Public survey polls designed to get the opinions of doctors have consistently shown that most physicians strongly opposed the transformation. Nearly half of doctors reportedly would have chosen a different profession or stopped practicing medicine if they had known of the pending regulations.

As many political analysts might have expected, these survey results put fire in the eyes of political cronies who support the Act. These individuals complained that such findings were partisan and distorted for political reasons.

Amid such controversy, key questions remain for both sides to consider. Most notably, why would physicians be happy with a bureaucracy that continually strives to limit their incomes? Why should they be pleased with excessive regulations and bureaucratic paperwork that ultimately increases operational costs?

To say that an overwhelming amount of doctors are universally pleased by Obamacare is tantamount to proclaiming that they're delighted by having their incomes slashed as the government dictates how they must treat specific patient conditions.

Required Changes in Care and Services

The labyrinth of confusing and overly abundant changes also will keep physicians and patients scrambling to qualify for numerous changes to the United States' healthcare infrastructure. Among them:

In-home care: Until now Medicare has never provided long-term health care, a service that had instead been handled by Medicaid at nursing homes or assisted-living facilities. Now Medicaid will surge into in-home care, thereby putting pressure on seniors to stay out of professional nursing homes—especially facilities considered by the government as expensive. The key question here remains unanswered: Will senior patients who agree to stay at home receive better or worse medical care?

Blending services: The neediest patients to treat as an overall group have been people who simultaneously use Medicare for health coverage and also Medicaid for expenses other than health care—such as nursing home stays. According to some estimates for every $100 spent on these "duel-eligible" individuals benefiting from Medicaid and Medicare, the cost is only $25 for "non-duals" served by only one program. The new rules will seek to rectify this by having the Department of Health and Human Services grow the bureaucracy, creating the Federal Coordinated Healthcare Office. The new division is supposed to cut red tape between Medicaid and Medicare. Critics worry that such improvements would be improbable or unlikely because each agency still has its own cumbersome and seemingly unbendable rules.

State bureaucracies: State governments will have to grow in order to fulfill new regulatory mandates for the required monitoring of nursing homes. State-run Websites will have to give specific information on such operations. To protect the interests of people who live in such facilities, the Act requires such operations to: publicly reveal specifics of operations including their employees' criminal records; reveal the identities of their owners so that residents will know where to complain; give residents at least 60 days notice before any planned closure; and develop ethical standards before publicly revealing whether those criteria have been met in order to discourage criminal conduct while cutting down on inadequate care. In addition, at its Web page, Medicare. gov, will post new information on how well nursing homes have performed.

Welcome to the Nanny State

Medicare and Medicaid each will eliminate co-pay requirements for certain pre-approved, government-authorized medical tests that could detect potential long-term health issues. This will be done partly as a way to encourage participants to take better care of themselves. The goal here is to reduce the lifetime health care costs of participants. But this new testing could ultimately pump up overall expenses. That's because many tests likely will detect an individual's health issues for the first time. Such diagnosis could ultimately increase all health care spending.

Among other potential healthcare or expense issues that could potentially erupt as a result of the new rules:

Nanny state: The list of requirements stemming directly or indirectly from Obamacare impact everything from restaurants to medical facilities. A "nanny-state" mindset began to take over in phases starting in 2011. The politicians had decided that the state and federal governments needed to dictate health matters to the general public. Big government essentially started to force-feed to the general public propaganda about calories, nutritional content and health maintenance procedures.

Restaurants: Starting in 2011, per-meal or per-item calorie totals and nutritional information needed to be posted on menus at restaurant chains with more than 19 facilities. The regulations became so outlandish that even vending machines that dispense snacks were required to post such nutritional information.

State-by-state inefficiencies: A state could potentially generate a 1-percent jump in how much it receives in federal assistance. Such revenue increases would be granted only in instances where the state has eliminated certain co-pays and given Medicaid recipients coverage for preventative procedures that the federal government wants patients to get. The federal government's goal is to motivate states to participate in preventative procedures. Yet this process ultimately could generate increases in overall costs.

Pro-active Medicare efforts: Seniors using Medicare will be encouraged to take a similar pro-active stance on their own health care. The government will urge them to undergo medical tests with no co-payments required for procedures that bureaucrats have approved. Doctors of these recipients will be encouraged to work with these patients individually in developing customized prevention plans.

Business forced to participate: The overall strategy of pushing the public to get preventative tests will extend beyond Medicare and Medicaid. The Act will guarantee that all Americans have access to certain preventative tests that bureaucrats have approved. In many instances specific tests will be recommended by federal workers or people who lack medical education before being appointed to regulatory panels. The new rules essentially will make employers the "big brothers" of their workers. Is this an invasion of a worker's privacy? Whatever the answer, the law will allow employers to give financial rewards to each worker who strives to become healthier. Complicating this issue, employers will be barred from using these criteria to discriminate against workers with pre-existing medical conditions or individuals who are unable to "reasonably" meet the conditions of improving their own health. Insurance plans will be set up as a guideline for the entire workforce of an employer.

Pilot programs: During 2014, Obamacare will launch numerous pilot programs in at least 10 states, an initial phase to determine the effectiveness of similar health insurance programs that encourage pro-active wellness efforts. A maze of bureaucrats without any medical education or experience will determine if the pilot program has been effective. Similar programs likely will start spreading to other states in 2017 if these political-crony panelists rule that the goal of increasing efficiencies has been achieved.

.

Accountable Care Organizations

All-out socialism will reach new heights throughout American society as the Act requires governments to launch "accountable care organizations" or ACOs.

Medical professionals will essentially work together in groups as "teams," who must treat all patients even those suffering from severe pre-existing medical conditions.

Huge teams of home-care providers, doctors and medical facilities including hospitals will work together. Patients who choose to participate are supposed to receive continuous care that is considered "comprehensive" or all-encompassing.

In a "grind-them-out system," doctors and hospitals will not be paid directly on a scale hinged to the quality of service, but rather the sheer numbers of patients. Thus, a doctor who sees one patient every ten minutes will earn far more than a physician who treats just one person every hour.

As a result a doctor who simply writes out a quick drug prescription after a brief chat with each patient will earn far more than physicians who actually spend substantial high-quality time to carefully diagnose a patient.

Eager to sidestep any potential criticisms, people who designed this goofy process also created a three-year test system that began in January 2012. This pilot program included a bonus system based on the supposed "quality" of care. Bonuses will be given only in instances where overall expenses are below pre-set money totals.

Once again, bureaucrats at the U.S. Department of Health and Human Services will make this determination. The goal was to give treatment "teams" financial incentives for their success in minimizing expenses by cooperating with each other.

Obamacare opponents who dislike this non-competitive strategy need to accept the fact that such teams might eventually permeate the U.S. medical industry as originally envisioned by people who created the Act.

Standardized Universal Medicine

The long-term strategy of these "accountable care organizations" is to demolish and obliterate today's entire fragmented U.S. medical infrastructure.

Supporters of Obamacare insist that once firmly set into place on a widespread scale the ACOs will dramatically increase the efficiency of the United States healthcare system. Under this so-called utopian society all health care professionals will efficiently and harmoniously work together in teams of hospitals, specialists and doctors.

To the contrary, the Act's opponents argue that these teams will actually wipe out competition. The result would be a system where patents are collectively treated like cattle marching into a stockyard. Under this line of thinking a patient would wait for weeks, months or even years just to see a doctor, the eventual visit lasting only a few minutes.

Some analysts say that the ACOs will not blossom on a widespread scale until perhaps 2017 and beyond, well after the state-run exchanges strengthen and achieve at least some degree of efficiency. Like the exchanges, ACOs eventually would serve as centralized services.

Numerous observers prefer to stop short of calling this "socialized" medicine, while others argue to the contrary. The first phase involved ACOs organized in conjunction with Medicare are already being set up to serve at least 2.4 million patients. Ideally, the federal government would not lead the way in this regard, but rather private industry.

Sporadic news reports indicated that various private insurance companies had started organizing ACOs by mid-2012. Left with no other choice but to follow the societal change sparked by Obamacare, hospitals and physicians groups started launching or clinging onto these unique new ventures as well.

.

James W. Forsythe, M.D., H.M.D.

Another Bureaucratic Phrase Emerged

Even more requirements emerged, as if these details weren't already enough to confuse average consumers and highly educated doctors. The new rules created another goofy, cumbersome term: "comparative effectiveness research." This is the catch-phrase referring to when bureaucrats analyze nationwide and statewide health care industry and insurance industry data to:

Fixes: Determine where to improve the system.

Savings: Develop ways to cut costs.

This "comparative effective research" objective likely will generate just as many problems as the process eventually solves.

Streams of bureaucrats and high-paid consultants will make a full-time living compiling these reports. Developing white papers and recommendations that likely will "never see the light of day," these research efforts will result from or depend on high-paid consultants, seminars, white papers, "think tanks," and so-called academics with little or no real-world experience.

If history is any indication of potential future results, then these very panels and think tanks are likely to generate confusion. Even casual observers might wonder if political affiliations and business alliances would weigh heavily on the panels' recommendations to the detriment of the general public.

The Greasy Hands of Big Government

Proponents of Obamacare often argue that the Act actually keeps the government out of the health care business—with hands-on work handled by physicians, medical facilities, hospitals and insurance providers. But even a casual review shows that the opposite is true. The Act puts the greasy hands of big government directly into the actions of hospitals and doctors as well. Among just some of the many examples:

Hospitals: Obamacare punishes hospitals by inflicting

strict financial penalties on such facilities that re-admit excessive numbers of Medicare patients within 30 days after those people are discharged. Critics claim that about one out of very five Medicare patients discharged from hospitals is soon re-admitted because they were discharged too soon. The unnecessary discharging and readmission of Medicare patients supposedly costs the government billions of dollars. Once again, government bureaucrats will scour data to identify which hospitals that the government will punish. The officials then would lower the money that "offending facilities" receive for Medicare. Even before imposing the penalties government officials do not yet know if the punishments will reverse the problem. Some hospitals will be exempt from potential penalties, particularly facilities in specified rural areas or within inner-city neighborhoods where the hospitals are the only providers.

Home: A highly ambitious aspect of Obamacare will bring health care services directly into the homes of needy Medicare recipients. Dubbed the "independence at home" program, this will involve teams of health care professionals collectively working to help patients, lower hospital readmissions and minimize fees. This so-called "demonstration" is geared toward Medicare percipients who suffer from numerous chronic ailments that cost the most money. In the "perfect world" envisioned by bureaucrats without medical training, at peak efficiency the program would literally take the human touch out of health care. When under the home-care program, a patient's vital signs such as blood pressure and heart rates would be monitored remotely via computers. This, in turn, would minimize the need for highly trained and continuously working health care professionals—at least from the view of bureaucrats without medical experience.

Ludicrous bureaucracy: Some cronies for the Obama administration have actually blamed patients for increasing health care costs. Such over-the-top criticisms blame people for unnecessarily visiting doctors too often, demanding costly treatments, and visiting specialists that they do not need. These political cronies, including a healthcare advisor to President Obama, even blast patients for supposedly wanting unnecessary, expensive hospital rooms that they should avoid. Obamacare supporters also blame doctors for excessively participating in a fee-for-service system that patients use far too much. The critics blame physicians for ordering more tests and more return visits than the patients apparently need, perhaps in part as a protective measure against potential frivolous malpractice lawsuits.

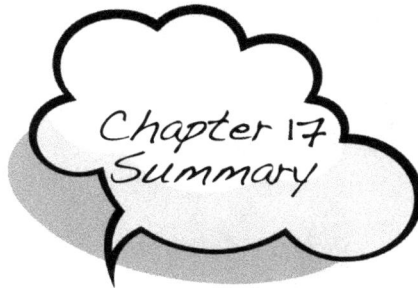

Chapter 17 Summary

Obamacare has sparked an out-of-control "nanny-state" bureaucracy that has pushed the government's hands into the USA's restaurants and health care infrastructure. Bureaucrats with no medical experience are dictating specifics of how and when citizens will receive health care—if at all. Measures and procedures designed to boost preventative care might actually increase overall medical costs. A system designed to enable the neediest Medicare recipients with multiple chronic conditions to remain at home will take the human touch out of healthcare. When entering the government's "independence at home" program, those patients will be monitored by robotic electronic machines that continually check the person's vital signs—the results sent to health care professionals via the Internet or high-tech communication devices. Bureaucratic panels comprised primarily of people with no medical training will work continuously in "think tanks" in an effort to cut health care costs while striving to increase efficiency. Starting a long-term strategy that many critics label as a precursor to inefficient socialized medicine, the government will steadily launch "accountable care organizations" or ACOs. These organizations will have teams of doctors, hospitals and health care facilities working together to treat large groups of individuals. Meantime, the government will impose strict penalties on hospitals that bureaucrats believe have prematurely discharged too many Medicare patients.

18
Obamacare Survival Tips

Since there is no escaping Obamacare, consumers nationwide need to follow these urgent tips in order to reap the most lucrative benefits from the program, and also to glide as easily as possible through the maze of bureaucratic rules:

Tip No. 1: Many U.S. taxpayers will qualify for government subsidies that help pay for their health insurance policies. So, check with your state-run exchange or the federally operated exchange for your state to see if you qualify. On a sliding scale, the federal government will pay up to 100 percent of these costs for individuals. You can only qualify for subsidies if your annual income as an individual or as a family is less than four times the federal poverty level. Under that rate, as of 2012 the maximum federal poverty level at four times the rate was $45,000 for an individual and $91,200 for a four-person family. When purchasing through an exchange, be sure to only buy a policy that has been officially authorized as qualified by the federal government.

Tip No. 2: For individuals or families with incomes too high to qualify for subsidies, options that might help "cope" with Obamacare include getting another job in order to help pay for mandatory insurance, or actually striving to earn less in order to become qualified for government subsidies. When considering these options, remember to check the charts within your state's official exchange in order to verify the subsidy qualification levels of a family the size of yours.

Tip No. 3: Check the possibility of applying to become a Medicaid recipient if you are not already benefiting from that federally funded program. Only low-income individuals or needy families can qualify. Yet Obamacare is widening the eligibility process. Until now, according to federal officials, millions of Americans had previously been unaware of the fact that they could qualify for Medicaid. Thus, streams of people will learn about the Medicaid program for the first time and start benefiting from this system, which requires no out-of-pocket payments from participants.

Tip No. 4: Obey all laws required by the Affordable Health Care Act. In essence, this means that you should never intentionally lie about your income level when completing your IRS forms, or when submitting applications for Medicaid or for federal subsidies while applying for policies. Criminal penalties for those who intentionally submit incorrect information can be severe. The IRS will have many thousands of new employees assigned to review tax forms in order to ensure that taxpayers submit correct information.

Tip No. 5: Avoid getting a new job from an employer that requires that you use its employer-funded health insurance policies if you have already applied for a federal subsidy. Some analysts say this strategy is particularly essential for married individuals or if they have children. Some bureaucrats and consultants claim that people cannot qualify for subsidies if their employer offers health insurance. However, you should also remember that an employer technically cannot force you to participate in a policy that it provides. And employers will be fined up to $2,000 for each instance where an employee voluntarily chooses to purchase his or her own health insurance in cases where the worker could be using employer-funded policies. In addition, remember that employers that offer insurance to workers are not required to make those policies affordable for families—but those policies must be affordable to an individual worker.

Tip No. 6: Unmarried adults who live with a person that

they love should consider avoiding any wedding vows, at least according to some analysts. Even if they file their taxes separately, married people will have to legally list their combined family incomes when applying for government subsidies. Under the federal poverty level listings of 2012 an unmarried individual earning $43,000 would qualify for at least some government assistance. But if that same individual were married to a person who earns $72,000, the potential applicant who earns $43,000 would not qualify for subsidies. Thus, Obamacare will be punishing many married people. This brings up the question of whether some married couples will start getting divorced while still intending to live together, legally ending their marital bond in order to qualify for subsidies.

Tip No. 7: Refuse to accept substantial raises from your employer until after checking with an experienced and highly educated financial advisor. Determine if the planned raise would disqualify you from receiving any federal subsidy that you received before such a planned income increase.

Tip No. 8: Carefully watch the summer or part-time job incomes of your dependent children. If those youngsters or young adults earn too much, you might become disqualified from eligibility for subsidies as a family. Children or young adults under age 26 might become encouraged to avoid part-time work in instances where their married parents' combined income levels are near the maximum federal poverty level.

Tip No. 9: Unless absolutely necessary, avoid paying any individual mandate penalties imposed on taxpayers who refuse to or fail to get health insurance policies. People who already have insurance policies listed as acceptable by the federal government should not have to worry about fulfilling such requirements. People who do not have policies should first check whether they would qualify for Medicaid. Individuals over 64 years old already covered by Medicare also do not need to worry. Taxpayers who refuse to or fail to buy policies—and don't have coverage through employers,

Medicaid or Medicare—will be fined on a sliding scale, depending on the year of the infraction. Those who pay fines will receive nothing in return for those expenditures. By purchasing policies they would at least get something. Taxpayers who choose to be fined for personal reasons should first determine whether the IRS is actually imposing the penalties before actually writing a check to the government.

Tip No. 10: People who retired early before age 65 should expect to lose the insurance that has been provided by their former employers. Analysts expect numerous companies to stop getting insurance for their retired ex-employees who had qualified for such coverage in their early-retirement plans. Some companies will attempt to justify such decisions because the exchanges likely will provide coverage at lower rates than if the corporations purchased the policies. All these changes would start during 2014. Early retirees who find themselves in this predicament likely will have to shop for policies via the exchanges.

Tip No. 11: Workers whose employers supply health insurance should check with the companies to see if the businesses provide rewards to those who maintain good health. Obamacare enables employers to get insurance policies that offer such incentives. In instances where such programs exist, employees who achieve certain standards of wellness could qualify for lower co-pays and lower premiums than their co-workers. If your employer offers such a program, take decisive action if necessary to improve your health in order to meet certain standards set by the policies. Such criteria might range from maintaining an ideal body weight to lowering blood pressure to healthful levels. Employees who fail to take such measures might end up paying up to 50 percent more than their co-workers for insurance policies. In addition, employees under such programs can consider asking for an exemption to opt-out of the health-maintenance system if believing they could never meet the so-called "good-health" standards.

Tip No. 12: Until Obamacare, people had been able to pay for over-the-counter drugs such as Tylenol by using funds from their Flexible Spending Accounts or their Health Savings accounts. But Obamacare prohibits such a process. Now people can only use such funds for drug purchases in instances where they get a prescription from a licensed doctor. Thus, consumers who have previously used such a process when purchasing non-prescription drugs should now plan ahead in order to get prescriptions for such pharmaceuticals.

Tip No. 13: Medicare recipients who have been using Medicare Advantage benefits from private providers should look for different choices. Many seniors have relied on such programs. But through the early 2020s Obamacare is expected to chip away at the federal government's Medicare Advantage budget. Thus, in order to ensure that they have enough supplemental coverage, seniors using Medicare Advantage will have to look for alternatives.

Tip No. 14: Prior to January 2014, adults considered as "high risks" because they have pre-existing health conditions can apply to enter a temporary insurance pool for such individuals. Until then, insurance companies will not be required to sell policies to adults with such conditions. (The insurance companies must grant such policies beginning in 2014.) In September 2010 Obamacare started requiring insurance companies to provide such policies for children. Yet many greedy insurance companies stopped issuing child-only policies in order to avoid such expenses. The firms no longer will be able to sidestep such costs starting January 1, 2014.

Tip No. 15: Couples who earn more than $250,000 and individuals with incomes greater than $200,000 need to know that Obamacare has targeted them as a primary revenue source for growing the government's healthcare bureaucracy. Such taxpayers will be stuck with higher federal tax bills in order to help augment the government's health care infrastructure expansion. Such taxes will stem in part from investment income and hospital insurance. Such individuals likely will get stuck paying more in taxes than they had been prior to Obamacare. Analysts say that any attempts to legally avoid these tax increases will become extremely difficult. Even so, such people should talk with their accountants or tax advisors to determine if there is a legal way for them to approach this issue.

Tip No. 16: Taxpayers at all income levels should strive to stay informed on Obamacare issues. Although Obamacare is unlikely to be repealed any time soon, consumers should remain aware that virtually all laws are continually modified. The details found in this book were in force as of 2013. But at least some changes are likely over time. As a result, the author of this publication maintains an eBook continually updated every six months to 12 months. It's available via the following Web link: **ObaminableCare.com**.

Tip No. 17: Owners of small businesses should check with their accountants or financial advisors in order to determine if required Obamacare provisions would make growing the company unfeasible. Obamacare provides tax credit incentives to small companies with less than 26 employees. Expanding a business might prove extremely damaging to the venture, depending on its own financing, needs and resources—when collectively considered in conjunction with the Act's rules imposed on larger companies.

Tip No. 18: Consumers should expect Obamacare to result in higher costs for a wide variety of items that they want to purchase, everything from food at grocery stores to fast-food restaurants such as pizza services. John Schnatter, CEO of the Papa John's pizza business, has estimated that the Affordable Health Care Act will result in price increases there from 11 cents to 14 cents per pizza. The owners of other huge nationwide businesses have given similar forecasts, complaining that their operations will need to pass higher health insurance costs on to consumers. If this scenario plays out as some business leaders predict, consumers will need to tighten their financial belts in order to help pay for Obamacare.

Tip No. 19: Many analysts also fear that cash-strapped state governments nationwide will be forced to raise taxes in order to cover their Medicaid expansion and insurance exchange operations fees. Thus, many taxpayers should expect to get gouged even more by increasingly bloated state and local governments. When and if such tax increases click into gear taxpayers should expect to have even less "spend-able" personal income. In summary, "you should save more so that you can give all that cash to the government."

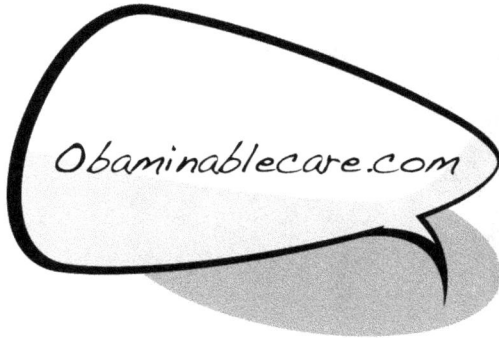

Obaminablecare.com

Medical payroll tax: Single people earning more than $200,000 and married couples earning more than $250,000 are getting slammed with $86.8 billion in Medicare payroll taxes.

19

Hidden Obamacare Taxes

Obamacare is loaded with little-known, clandestine taxes that the general public lacks any knowledge about, fees that likely would anger many Americans if they knew the truth. Among some of the most destructive new taxes:

2010

Indoor tanning tax: This began July 10, 2010, slapping $2.7 billion in annual fees on indoor tanning salons.

Shield tax hikes on Blue Cross/Blue Shield: these services that enjoyed deductions under previous law got slammed with $400 million in new fees starting in January 2010. The new regulation allows special tax deductions in cases where only 85 percent of premiums go toward clinical services.

Innovator drug companies' tax: Starting in January 2010, these fees jumped an estimated $22.2 billion, hooked on a relative scale of annual sales.

Bio-fuel tax: Labeled by bureaucrats as the "black liquor" tax, starting in 2010 this imposed a $23.6 billion tax hike on bio-fuels.

IRS cruelty: Obamacare enables, encourages and clears the way for the IRS to arbitrarily and at its own discretion hike taxes by $4.5 billion. A bureaucratic term called the "economic substance doctrine" would allow the Internal Revenue Service to rule that certain tax deductions—which previously would have been deemed legal—can no longer be considered as having "substance."

Punish charitable hospitals: When bureaucrats rule that a charitable hospital has failed to meet "community health assessment needs," the institutions will have to pay $50,000 penalties.

2011

Health Savings Accounts: The federal HAS started imposing $1.4 billion in taxes, increasing penalties for early withdrawls from such accounts to 20 percent—doubling the previous 10-percent fees.

Penalize savings: Swiping $5 billion in benefits from consumers, starting in January 2011, the federal government started penalizing health savings accounts, health reimbursements and flexible-spending accounts.

2013

Investment Income Surtax: Hardworking and financially successful Americans were slapped with $123 billion in new taxes on their investment income. Those funds were earmarked to provide no-fee Obamacare medical services for low-income Americans.

Three-year-fee: A total $25 billion will be collected in temporary three-year fees of $63 per person, to cover fees of people with pre-existing medical conditions.

Compensation deductions: Starting in January 2013, a total $600 million would be raised, to cover the compensation deductions would reach $500,000 per worker—down from the previous $1 million.

Remove Tax Deductions: This would remove $4.5 billion from the deductions on taxes, instances where companies provide retired employees with drug coverage.

Spending caps: Starting in January 2013, Obamacare limited to $2,500 the amount that consumers could pay or use toward Flexible Spending Accounts geared toward health care. The previous rules had no limit on such spending, which cover everything from the special needs of children to dependant care and medical expenses.

Taxes on high medical bills: Starting in January 2013, the IRS increased to 10 percent of adjusted gross income from the previous 7.5 percent the threshold at which taxpayers could begin deducting medical expenses. As a result, a decreased number of taxpayers will qualify for such deductions.

Medical device manufacturers: Bowing to public sentiment and a push by health industry lobbyists, in the spring of 2013 the U.S. Senate took an initial step in eliminating taxes that would have been imposed in January of that year. The new rule, eventually repealed by Congress, would impose $20 billion in taxes on the medical device manufacturing industry—which employs more than a third of a million people at 6,000 facilities nationwide.

Medical payroll tax: Single people earning more than $200,000 and married couples earning more than $250,000 are getting slammed with $86.8 billion in Medicare payroll taxes.

2014

Bureaucrats estimate that mandatory insurance imposed on companies and individuals will cost at least $65 billion.

Health insurers: Starting in January 2014, new taxes on health insurers, generating an estimated $60.1 billion and imposed on insurance companies earning at least $50 million in profits.

Industry fines: Companies with more than 49 employees will have to pay an additional non-deductible tax of $2,000 in fines for each instance where a full-time employee is not offered health care coverage—and the worker qualifies for a health-tax credit.

Excise tax: Labeled by bureaucrats as an "individual mandate excise tax," for the first time in U.S. history individual taxpayers will have to pay fees to the IRS for instances where these individuals fail to or refuse to buy federally prescribed health insurance policies. On a sliding scale steadily increasing over a period of years, the fees will reach 2.5 percent of the individual's personal income or $695, whichever is greater.

2018
"Cadillac" Health Insurance Plans: Financially successful individuals who independently choose to buy top-of-the-line health insurance policies will be forced to pay a whopping 40-percent excise tax. Bureaucrats estimate this will generate $32 billion in annual revenue for the federal government. These will impact the most expensive health insurance plans that cost $10,200 or more for individuals and at least $27,500 for families.)

.

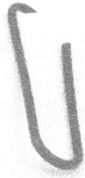

Notes!!

Chapter 1

The Internal Revenue Code, Pub. L 111-148, listed in
scattered sections
National Institutes of Health Fact Sheets
"The Wall Street Journal," various news reports
"JacksonFreePress.com," report of February 11, 2013
"RealClearPolitics.com," report of February 7, 2013
realclearpolitics.com/articles/2013/02/07/cbo_is_
increasingly_skeptical_about_obamacare_116951.html
National Journal, as cited in Real Clear Politics article

Chapter 2

Fox News
San Francisco Examiner online
The Heritage Foundation online
San Jose Mercury News

Chapter 3

✓ Singhal, "How U.S. Health Care Health Care Reform Will Effect Employee Benefits

Chapter 4

✓ The Affordable Health Care Act

Chapter 5

✓ New York Post
nypost.com/p/news/opinion/opedcolumnists/
how_obamacare_destroys_your_privacy_
zItwZSGoI661FeB1iC5POI
USA Today column, Dec. 6, 2012, usatoday.com/story/
opinion/2012/12/06/column-potential-obamacare-privacy-
nightmare/1752211/
http://www.heritage.org/research/reports/2010/04/
obamacare-impact-on-taxpayers

Chapter 7

✓ The Heritage Foundation
http://www.aamc.org/newsroom/pressrel/2010/100510f.htm
http://www.heritage.org/Research/Reports/2006/12/The-Urgent-
Need-to-Reform-Medicares-Physician-Payment-System

Chapter 8

✓ http://blogs.ajc.com/kyle-wingfield/2012/11/01/revealed-
what-the-irs-form-for-obamacare-might-look-like/

Chapter 9

✓ Law.com, article published February 12, 2013, by Wayne Jacobson

Chapter 10

✓ Foster, "Estimated Financial Effects;" Douglas Elmendorf, letter to Jeff Sessions, United States Senate, January 22, 2010

Chapter 14

✓ http://www.washingtonpost.com/blogs/wonkblog/wp/2013/02/18/its-official-the-feds-will-run-most-obamacare-exchanges/

Chapter 16

✓ http://www.denverpost.com/recommended/ci_13261279
World Health Organization
National Institutes of Health
http://www.nationalreview.com/articles/333535/how-s-obamacare-waiver-workin-out-ya-michelle-malkin

Chapter 17

✓ http://www.dickmorris.com/review-of-obamacare-survival-guide/

About the Author

James W. Forsythe, M.D., H.M.D., has long been considered one of the most respected physicians in the United States, particularly for his treatment of cancer and the legal use of human growth hormone. In the mid-1960s, Dr. Forsythe graduated with honors from University California at Berkeley and earned his Medical Degree from University of California, San Francisco, before spending two years residency in Pathology at Tripler Army Hospital, Honolulu. After a tour of duty in Vietnam, he returned to San Francisco and completed an internal medicine residency and an oncology fellowship. He is also a world-renowned speaker and author. He has co-authored, been mentioned in and/or written chapters in bestsellers. To name a few: "An Alternative Medicine Definitive Guide to Cancer;" "Knockout, Interviews with Doctors who are Curing Cancer" Suzanne Somers' number one bestseller; "The Ultimate Guide To Natural Health, Quick Reference A-Z Directory of Natural Remedies for Diseases and Ailments;" "Anti-Aging Cures;" "The Healing Power of Sleep;" "Outsmart Your Cancer: Alternative Non-Toxic Treatments That Work" and "Compassionate Oncology ~ What Conventional Cancer Specialists Don't Want You To Know;" and "Obaminable Care," "Complete Pain," "Natural Pain Killers," and "Your Secret to the Fountain of Youth ~ What They Don't Want You to Know About HGH Human Growth Hormone," "Take Control of Your Cancer," and the "Emergency Radiation Medical Handbook."

Contact Information

Century Wellness Clinic, 521 Hammill Lane
Reno, NV, 89511
(775) 827-0707
RenoWellnessDr@Yahoo.com

www.ingramcontent.com/pod-product-compliance
Lightning Source LLC
Chambersburg PA
CBHW070802290326
41931CB00011BA/2106